ch2

Health Information Management

Health Information Management

Principles and Organization for Health Information Services

FIFTH EDITION

MARGARET A. SKURKA

Editor

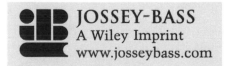

JOSSEY-BASS
A Wiley Imprint
www.josseybass.com

Health Forum, Inc.
An American Hospital Association Company
CHICAGO

Published by Jossey-Bass
A Wiley Imprint
989 Market Street, San Francisco, CA 94103-1741   www.josseybass.com

Jossey-Bass books and products are available through most bookstores. To contact Jossey-Bass directly call our Customer Care Department within the U.S. at 800-956-7739, outside the U.S. at 317-572-3986 or fax 317-572-4002.

Jossey-Bass also publishes its books in a variety of electronic formats. Some content that appears in print may not be available in electronic books.

Library of Congress Cataloging-in-Publication Data
Health information management : principles and organization for health record services / edited by Margaret Skurka.—5th ed.
    p. ; cm.
Rev. ed. of: Health information management / Margaret A. Skurka. Rev. ed. c1998.
Includes bibliographical references and index.
  ISBN 0-7879-5977-4 (alk. paper)
  1. Medical records—Management. 2. Information storage and retrieval systems—Hospital.
  [DNLM: 1. Medical Records. 2. Hospital Information Systems. 3. Medical Records Department, Hospital—organization & administration. WX173 H4334 2002] I. Skurka, Margaret Flettre.
  RA976 .S568 2002
  651.5'04261—dc21   2002153516

Printed in the United States of America
FIFTH EDITION
PB Printing   10 9 8 7 6 5 4 3 2 1

CONTENTS

PREFACE

H ealth Information Management: Principles and Organization for Health Information Services, Fifth Edition, recognizes the continuing need for guidance in developing efficient health information management (HIM) systems for health care institutions. This important revision of the 1998 edition is designed to capture the significant changes in the HIM field and profession in recent years.

The first edition of this book was published in 1984, and it replaced *Medical Record Departments in Hospitals: Guide to Organization,* which had originally been published by the American Hospital Association in 1962 and revised in 1972. Second and third editions of the book were published in 1988 and 1994, respectively, under the title *Organization of Medical Record Departments in Hospitals.*

This book serves as a comprehensive general reference to patient records and HIM. It is useful to a health care institution's chief executive, chief operating and financial officers, and information systems technology personnel. It is also essential reading for health professionals who need a general overview and understanding of HIM practices. The text covers appropriate information for faculty and students in health information administration and technology educational programs, and it serves as an introduction to HIM practices and issues for information systems (sometimes called informatics or information technology) programs. In addition, individuals in smaller health care institutions will find this book useful in applying the basic principles of HIM. As the appropriate application of these basic principles requires a careful analysis of the individual health care institution's needs, various operations in HIM are discussed herein.

The health care industry continues to undergo change, and the technology used in managing health information has experienced very rapid change. The electronic patient record is in place in many institutions, and the Internet has had a significant impact. The HIM managers of the future will manage data electronically, oversee document and repository systems, coordinate patient information, secure all electronically maintained information under HIPAA (Health Insurance and Accountability Act), supply senior management with information for decision making and strategy development, ensure data quality, and direct enterprise- or facilitywide HIM departments.

Throughout this book, the term *health information management* will be used to encompass both the registered health information administrator (RHIA) and the registered health information technician (RHIT), because professionals at both levels hold a variety of positions within the discipline. Specific references are made to the department director as a "HIM manager" who may be an RHIA or an RHIT. Because *health record* and *health information management* have almost completely replaced *medical record* and *medical record management,* only the current terminology will be used in this book.

The American Health Information Management Association (AHIMA) has more than 42,000 members. In addition to the credentialing of RHIAs and RHITs, the organization sponsors examinations leading to the advanced coding credentials of CCS (certified coding specialist) and CCS-P (certified coding specialist-physician). Entry-level certification as a CCA (certified coding associate) is also available, as is certification in the field of health care privacy as a CHP (certification in health care privacy). Together, all these individuals provide the expertise necessary to develop and maintain the health information systems necessary in this new millennium.

ACKNOWLEDGMENTS

A significant thanks goes out to my contributing authors for this edition of *Health Information Management: Principles and Organization for Health Information Services*. Without their assistance, this work would not have been possible. They each contributed their experience in the specific areas of health information management in which they work, which gives this text a real hands-on feel. They were timely and on point—consistently. Thank you Nancy Coffman-Kadish, Elizabeth Contant, Linda Kiger, Desla Mancilla, and Faye Pickett.

A special thank-you goes to my family, as always—husband Richard and children Erik, Kirstin, and Erin—who again, during my fifth revision of this work, showed patience, understanding, and support for long hours and weekend time spent at the computer. They've always understood and accepted my intensity and commitment with regard to this profession, and for that I am grateful. This book is dedicated to them and to my very wonderful parents, Edward and Ella Flettre Galvanek. They instilled in me both a strong work ethic and an appreciation of life.

THE EDITOR

Margaret A. Skurka, MS, RHIA, CCS, is professor and director of the Health Information Management Programs at Indiana University Northwest in Gary. She received her baccalaureate in health information management from the University of Illinois and was awarded a master of science in education from Purdue University. Skurka is actively involved in the American Health Information Management Association, having served as national president in 2000. She served a six-year term on the board of directors. Skurka has served as an accreditation site surveyor, is a past president of the Indiana Health Information Management Association, and was named that association's distinguished member in 1987. She was named the Alumnus of the Year in the Allied Health Professions at the University of Illinois at Chicago in 2002. She is the author of many ICD-9-CM physician coding reference products. As a consultant, Skurka has worked for numerous physician practices, ambulatory care centers, and surgery centers and has conducted ICD-9-CM and CPT coding seminars across the nation.

THE CONTRIBUTORS

Nancy Coffman-Kadish, MS, RHIA, is a clinical assistant professor and the clinical coordinator of the Health Information Technology Program at Indiana University Northwest in Gary. She received her baccalaureate in health information administration from the College of St. Scholastica in Duluth, Minnesota, and a master's degree in education from Indiana University. She is also currently a consultant in various ambulatory care settings, including surgery centers and physician practices. She has been an HIM professional for nearly twenty-five years and has been active in professional association activities. She served as president of the Indiana Health Information Management Association and held various positions on the executive board. She has also served at the national level in the American Health Information Management Association.

Elizabeth A. Contant, MBA, RHIA, CCS-P, is the director of coding and reimbursement at DuPage Medical Group in Glen Ellyn, Illinois. She received her baccalaureate in health information management from the University of Illinois and earned a master of business administration from DePaul University in Chicago. She also earned her CCS-P (certified coding specialists-physician) certification from the American Health Information Management Association. She has extensive coding and compliance experience; she has presented ICD-9-CM and CPT/HCPCS coding audio seminars and has conducted workshops for various multispecialty physician groups in the Chicago area. Contant has served as guest faculty for the University of Illinois Health Information Administration Program.

Linda S. Kiger, MBA, RHIA, CPHQ, is director of quality management and privacy officer at St. Anthony Medical Center in Crown Point, Indiana. Her responsibilities and duties include performance improvement, infection control, HIPAA implementation and enforcement, privacy, and compliance; she serves as the accreditation and licensure survey coordinator. Kiger received her baccalaureate in health information management and her master's degree in business administration from Indiana University. Prior to assuming her current position, Kiger had many years of experience in the health information management profession, serving as a director of health information management, with responsibility for the medical staff office; she served as a clinical site supervisor. She is a registered health information administrator and also holds the credential of certified professional in health care quality.

Desla R. Mancilla, MPA, RHIA, is the information protection officer for the Community Healthcare System–Community Hospital in Munster, Indiana. She received her baccalaureate degree in health information administration from the College of St. Scholastica in Duluth, Minnesota, and a master's degree in public administration from Indiana University Northwest in Gary. Mancilla previously held the position of system analyst and electronic patient record system project manager at Community Hospital. She has served on a variety of committees at the national level for the American Health Information Management Association and served as president of the Indiana Health Information Management Association. Mancilla is a frequent speaker at regional and state meetings regarding HIPAA and patient privacy matters and has published several articles and chapters related to electronic patient record systems.

Faye Pickett, MPA, RHIA, was a clinical assistant professor in the School of Biomedical and Health Information Sciences, College of Applied Health Sciences, University of Illinois at Chicago. She was the recipient of the college's Excaliber Award for Teaching Excellence in 1999 and 2000. She received her baccalaureate in health information management from Stephens College and was awarded a master's in public health from Indiana University. Pickett is actively involved in the American Health Information Management Association, having served on its professional practice committee; she also served on the editorial review board for *In Confidence* and on several committees within the Long-Term Care Section. Pickett is the author of numerous articles and has served as a guest speaker to various organizations in the HIM field. She is currently spending time with her family at home.

Health Information Management

CHAPTER 1

Health Information Management and the Health Care Institution

Faye Pickett

The terms *medical record* and *health record* are sometimes used interchangeably in referring to the document that captures the health information of a patient. However, a distinction should be made between the two types of records. *Medical record* implies that physicians participate in and supervise the medical care provided to patients in health care institutions. *Health record* is a term that encompasses not only the record of medical care provided but also a listing of services provided by nonphysician health care practitioners. This accounting may include records of an individual's health status that are kept on file with an agency, third-party payer, non–health care institution, or even by the patient. Such health records may be used in health benefits administration, applications for insurance coverage, research studies, and employment records, as well as in social service plans for individual or family care.

As the health information management (HIM) profession shifts its focus from the hard-copy paper record to an electronic patient record, data elements become the critical component of the record. In the paper record, data elements were found on various forms. Because there are no forms in a true electronic patient record, these data elements convey the patient's encounter through computerized means.

The health record is a valuable tool in providing high-quality patient care, preventing disease, and promoting health. Health records assist the preparation of the health service statistics used to evaluate the efficiency and effectiveness of care and to substantiate the provision of patient care services and treatment. The health record supports medical education, health services, and clinical research, and it provides documentation for the reimbursement of expenditures for health care services. It is also used in developing public policy on health care, including regulation, legislation, accreditation, and health care reform.

The Joint Commission on Accreditation of Healthcare Organizations (JCAHO) is a voluntary organization that accredits hospitals. A hospital must demonstrate substantial overall compliance with the Joint Commission's standards for hospital operations. JCAHO also accredits other types of health care facilities such as long-term care, mental health, and ambulatory care.

The Commission on Accreditation of Rehabilitation Facilities (CARF) may accredit rehabilitation facilities. Included in both CARF and JCAHO standards are requirements for the maintenance and adequacy of health records. A facility may also be certified for Medicare and Medicaid reimbursement through federal regulations, as published by the Center for Medicare and Medicaid Services (CMS). Facilities should also be licensed by the state they are in. Directly or indirectly, the board of trustees, the CEO, the medical staff, and the HIM professional all share responsibility to meet these standards, regulations, and policies regarding the health record. This chapter provides an overview of each group's role in the creation, maintenance, and protection of health information to ensure that it is accurate, timely, and complete. (See Figure 1.1.)

RESPONSIBILITY OF THE BOARD OF TRUSTEES AND CEO FOR HIM

An institution's governing body, or board of trustees, typically comprises individuals who are recognized leaders in their field and have a responsible standing in the community. Trustees may be appointed or elected by the existing board or by the corporate office to serve for a specific term.

The board of trustees is responsible for establishing policy, maintaining high-quality patient care, and providing institutional management and planning for the health care institution. To fulfill its responsibilities, the board establishes mechanisms for performing necessary policymaking, planning, and administrative functions, including functions related to HIM. These mechanisms include appointment of a CEO, support for the medical staff in quality management, and creation of appropriate committees.

The board holds the CEO responsible for implementing established policies for the operation of the institution and for keeping the board well informed about day-to-day operations. The CEO is also responsible for informing the board about federal, state, and local events that may affect the planning and operation of the facility.

The board holds the medical staff responsible for the development, adoption, and periodic review of medical staff bylaws and rules and regulations that are consistent with the facility's policy. The medical staff, as well as the staffs of other departments, are required to implement and report on the activities and mechanisms for monitoring and evaluating the quality of patient care. The purpose of monitoring and evaluating is twofold: (1) to identify opportunities for improving patient care and (2) to identify and resolve patient care problems.

Although the board of trustees is ultimately responsible for the health care institution, the optimal operation of the facility requires the combined effort of the board, CEO, and medical staff. This is typically accomplished through the establishment of a joint committee to address activities and problems of mutual concern.

Figure 1.1. Responsibility for Health Information

Board of Trustees

- Corporate planning
- Maintaining quality care
- Establishing policymaking, planning, and administrative mechanisms
- Appointing the Chief Executive Officer
- Having ultimate responsibility for the health care institution

Chief Executive Officer

- Approving the budget for implementing systems for maintaining health information
- Providing direction, staffing, and facilities for HIM
- Enforcing information management regulations, policies, and standards
- Protecting health information
- Running day-to-day operations for the health care facility

Medical Staff

- Reviewing health information rules, regulations, policies, and standards
- Participating in decisions regarding health information systems format or forms content
- Specifying medical staff membership qualifications
- Delineating clinical privileges qualifications
- Authenticating medical record entries

HIM Department

- Maintaining a health information storage and retrieval system
- Preserving health information confidentiality, security, integrity, and access
- Coding and classifying health information
- Managing all patient health information
- Organizing, producing, and disseminating health information

Figure 1.1. Continued

HIM Professional

- Coordinating data collection
- Monitoring information integrity
- Ensuring access to health information by qualified individuals
- Organizing, analyzing, and evaluating health information
- Consulting on information management issues for other departments
- Compiling administrative and health statistics
- Coding diagnoses, therapies, and other procedures
- Inputting and retrieving health information
- Monitoring standards and regulations regarding information management

Maintenance and Protection of Health Information

The health record is maintained for the purpose of providing quality care. Proper maintenance of this health information serves the patient, health care professionals, and the facility. The CEO is responsible to the governing body for implementing a system for maintaining adequate health information, whether a hard-copy medical record or an electronic patient record. The CEO is also responsible for safeguarding the record and its content against loss, defacement, and unauthorized use. Federal regulations mandate the privacy and security of health information.

The CEO and the HIM Department

In addition to maintaining systems, the CEO is also accountable for the administrative functions of the institution and for delegating duties and responsibilities to subordinates. This management function includes providing the HIM department with proper direction, staffing, and facilities to perform all required functions. Therefore, it is important that the CEO know the skills and competencies of the HIM professional.

RESPONSIBILITY OF THE MEDICAL STAFF

A facility's bylaws, rules, and regulations dictate each medical staff member's responsibility for maintaining timely, accurate, and complete health records. The institution's CEO and its organized medical staff share the responsibility for ensuring that the facility's health records are complete and in accordance with the bylaws and rules and regulations for self-government approved by the board. Health record rules and regulations apply to the entire medical staff and should be uniformly enforced.

Medical staff should also actively participate in decisions regarding the maintenance of health information, including the format and design of the paper medical record or the information system in an electronic medical record. Members of the medical staff may participate in the medical record committees or forms committees.

Rule Compliance Review and Monitoring

As part of the health care facility's performance improvement activities, the medical staff is responsible for the regular review of all rules, regulations, and policies related to medical record requirements. A clinical pertinence documentation review consists of evaluating the completeness, adequacy, appropriateness, accuracy, and quality of documentation.

The objective of a review process is to ensure that each health record includes (1) sufficient documentation of the patient's condition, progress, and outcome of care, (2) documentation for the administration of tests and therapy as ordered, and (3) documentation for notification and acceptance in any transfer of patient responsibility from one physician to another. The review process should also consider the adequacy of the health record for the institution's performance improvement, utilization, and risk management activities. The standards of JCAHO imply that a quality improvement process is in place in all departments. Therefore, professionals from HIM, nursing services, medical staff, and all others involved in health record documentation should take part in the record review process.

Clinical Privileges and Credentialing

In keeping with JCAHO standards on the management of information services, as described in the *Accreditation Manual for Hospitals,* the medical staff is responsible for specifying its membership categories and delineating qualifications for the granting of clinical privileges. Physicians wishing to obtain privileges for a specific institution must apply for medical staff membership or clinical privileges. The granting of membership and privileges makes the affected individual responsible for adhering to the medical staff's existing rules and regulations for HIM. The exercise of clinical privileges within any department, if there are medical staff clinical departments, is subject to its rules and regulations and to the authority of the department chair. Although the medical staff bears overall responsibility for the quality of professional services provided by those who are granted clinical privileges, the final accountability lies with the governing board.

Responsibility of Other Health Care Professionals

The physician should complete several parts of the medical record, including the history and physical, discharge summary, physician's orders, and progress notes. In addition, other health care professionals provide services, and they must document those services in the medical record.

Nursing services, for example, document mostly through such means as nursing progress notes, graphic records, and medication records. Nurses may work with social workers in developing a discharge plan. Dietary services may document the patient's nutritional needs. In addition, therapies such as physical, occupational, or speech may be provided. Each one of these professionals contributes to the medical record through the provision of progress notes.

Entries must be authenticated and reviewed to ensure data quality. In addition, each professional has a role to play in maintaining the security of health information.

Authentication of Entries

To ensure that entries are authentic, they should be dated and signed by the author. Entries that require a countersignature by supervisors or attending medical staff members should be defined in the medical staff rules and regulations. Although state and federal regulations and agency standards should always be adhered to, authentication can generally be defined as a written signature or initials, electronic signature, or rubber-stamp signature.

When rubber-stamp signatures are authorized for use in authenticating entries, their use must be controlled. The individual whose signature is replicated on a stamp should place a signed statement on file in the administrative offices of the facility stating that he or she is the only one who has the stamp and is the only one who will use it.

FUNCTIONS OF THE HIM DEPARTMENT

The HIM department supports the facility's optimal standards for quality care and services by providing quality information. Its functions support the patient through the entire continuum of the patient's care. In addition, it supports administrative processes, billing through classification systems, medical education, research through data gathering and analysis, utilization, risk and quality management programs, legal requirements, data security, and release of information to authorized users.

THE HIM PROFESSIONAL

The HIM professional is the institution's specialist on managing and utilizing health care data. This professional often communicates with administration, financial services, and health care professionals to ensure that the data are timely, complete, valid, and secure.

Definition of Responsibilities

The American Health Information Management Association (AHIMA) is the professional association for HIM professionals. AHIMA states that one of the primary goals of the HIM professional is to enhance patient care through the provision of timely and relevant information.[1] This professional is the expert in managing medical records and information systems. AHIMA states that the HIM professional is uniquely qualified to

- Ensure that health information is complete and available to legitimate users
- Code and classify data for reimbursement
- Analyze information necessary for decision support
- Protect patient privacy and provide information security
- Enhance the quality of uses for data within health care
- Administer health information computer systems
- Comply with standards and regulations regarding health information
- Prepare health data for accreditation surveys
- Analyze clinical data for research and public policy

HIM professionals are responsible for securing, analyzing, managing, and integrating health information. This integration of health information has become an important function, as health care facilities focus on providing a continuum of care services to the patient. In this system, patients and their health information would easily move across several levels of care.

The information provided by HIM is used by health care professionals in making medical decisions and by the organization in making business decisions. As the expert, the HIM professional performs a variety of functions, including

- Compiling research and administrative statistics
- Coding, inputting, analyzing, and securing data
- Performing quality improvement studies
- Providing decision support services

This professional may also be responsible for maintaining indexes, such as the master patient index (MPI), which may be one of the most important tools because it identifies all of the patients who have received care at the facility.[2] Whatever the specific function, the HIM professional is responsible for maintaining the health information system, whether it is computerized or on paper.

In small facilities, the professional may be responsible for providing support services to medical staff. The HIM professional should be knowledgeable about current JCAHO standards and current state and federal requirements. The professional may serve on various committees within the organization. Such committees may include medical records, utilization management, and quality management.

Career Opportunities in HIM

Every organization involved in health and wellness needs professionals to manage information. Thus HIM professionals may work in a variety of settings, including[3]

- Hospitals
- Managed care organizations
- Long-term care facilities
- Behavioral health facilities
- Consulting and law firms
- Information systems vendors
- Ambulatory care facilities
- Rehabilitation centers
- Skilled nursing facilities
- Home care providers
- Government agencies
- Pharmaceutical companies

- Physician practices

- Insurance companies

As the dynamics of the health care industry continue to evolve, HIM professionals' roles may include health data management, service to the health care consumer, or information resource management.

Educational Requirements for HIM

Current baccalaureate-level educational requirements of health information administration programs accredited by the AHIMA Council on Accreditation require courses in the following content areas:

- Biomedical sciences, including anatomy, physiology, language of medicine, medical sciences, pharmacology
- Information technology
- Health care delivery systems
- Organization and supervision
- Quantitative methods and research
- Health care information requirements and standards
- Health care information systems
- Health data content and structure
- Clinical quality assessment and performance improvement
- Biomedical research support
- Health information services management

Expertise in the areas listed helps equip the graduate for the expanded HIM role that the professional will play in the future. After graduation from an accredited HIA program, the graduate becomes eligible to write the Registered Health Information Administration (RHIA) exam. Passage of this exam allows professionals to use the RHIA credentials after their name to illustrate their role as a HIM. The RHIA is required to maintain thirty continuing education hours every two years in order to maintain his or her credentials.

The curriculum for an accredited health information technology program is similar; it requires the following:

- Biomedical sciences, including anatomy, physiology, language of medicine, medical sciences, pharmacology
- Information technology
- Health data content
- Health care delivery systems
- Organization and supervision
- Health care statistics and data literacy
- Clinical quality assessment and performance improvement
- Clinical classification systems
- Reimbursement methodologies
- Legal and ethical issues

After graduation from an accredited HIT program, the graduate becomes eligible to write the registered health information technician (RHIT) exam. Passage of this exam allows the professional to use the credentials RHIT. The RHIT is required to maintain twenty continuing education hours every two years in order to maintain his or her credentials.

Mastery of these core contents, at either the baccalaureate or associate level, will help ensure that the graduate entering the profession possesses the entry-level competencies for success in the future. Some universities offer a graduate degree in health informatics, whose curriculum places a major emphasis on information systems.

In addition, the HIM professional may become certified in coding by passing the Certified Coding Specialist (CCS), Certified Coding Specialist–Physician-Based (CCS-P), or Certified Coding Associate (CCA) exams. Passage of the CCS exam demonstrates competency in coding and data quality and integrity, mainly in the hospital setting. The CCS-P exam also assesses proficiency in coding and data quality and integrity, but in physician-based settings rather than the hospital. The CCA exam was devised to serve as an entry-level exam for those just beginning their coding careers.

Since the assurance of privacy is vital to a health care institution, the HIM professional may also become Certified in Healthcare Privacy (CHP). Passage of this exam demonstrates proficiency in the designing and administering of privacy programs in various types of health care institutions.

Job Descriptions

Through managing health information, the professional contributes to the quality of care provided to the patient. Positions an HIM professional may hold include[4]

- HIM department director
- HIM system manager
- Data quality manager
- Information security officer
- HIM college instructor
- Consultant
- Health data analyst
- Insurance claims analyst
- Clinical coding specialist
- Physician practice manager
- Patient information coordinator
- Privacy officer
- Corporate compliance officer

HIM Department Director

As a department director, the HIM professional determines health information policies, budgets, and resources; acts as liaison with other departments, and evaluates employee performance. The managerial skills of the department director must include the ability to organize functions and workload for maximum productivity, provide overall direction to department personnel, assist members of the medical staff in carrying out their responsibilities relative to the health record, and adhere to the established policies, rules, and regulations of the institution.

The HIM director is responsible for investigating delays in the gathering of reports that are vital to the content and completeness of the record. Delays cause problems in continuing care and reimbursement and call for immediate attention. To avoid delays resulting from insufficient information, it is essential that the HIM department communicate with other departments in the institution. In fact, in some organizations the director may also be in charge of other departments such as admitting and utilization management.

Vision 2006 Roles

Vision 2006, developed in 1996, is the framework of the profession as promulgated by AHIMA.[5] Its purpose was to identify the strategic direction and roles of the future. These roles include the following:

- Managers of integrated systems
- Clinical data specialists
- Patient information coordinators
- Data quality managers, who ensure data integrity
- Data resource administrators
- Information security managers
- Research and decision support analysts

These roles were devised for the integration of technology into the health care industry. Over time these functions will evolve from department-based operations to an information environment as the documentation of health information moves from a paper record to a computerized patient record.

Health Insurance Portability and Accountability Act

The Health Insurance Portability and Accountability Act (HIPAA) was signed into law in 1996. Two major purposes of HIPAA are administrative simplification and data security. In December 2000, the Standards for Privacy of Individually Identifiable Health Information were released by the federal government. These standards require that facilities assign a privacy official to be responsible for the development and implementation of policies and procedures regarding privacy. HIM professionals are uniquely qualified to hold this position through their experience with maintaining confidentiality and access to health information (see AHIMA Position Statement: Privacy Officer Position, at the end of this book).

HIPAA also requires a corporate compliance program to ensure ethical business practices. Through their knowledge of coding, accurate documentation, and billing, the HIM professional is qualified to serve as the corporate compliance officer.[6]

Relationships with Other Departments

The HIM professional interacts with all of the departments and services that generate information to be included in individual patients' records. The HIM professional should therefore be familiar with the reporting systems and procedures used for generating reports in the diagnostic and therapeutic areas. In addition, the HIM professional often functions as a consultant for information systems in other areas of the organization. For example, the HIM professional may be called on to work with a department such as physical therapy to see what data elements they may want to use in an electronic medical record.

The quality of the patient record depends in part on the timeliness and meaningfulness of the content entered by all individuals who are given the authority and responsibility for documenting their participation in patient care. The usefulness of health information depends in part on the legibility of entries and on the ability to identify the individuals who have entered the information, whether manual or computerized. Illegible handwriting, poor form design, or inadequate safeguards and controls on data entry can create problems in using the health information for continuing care and data abstracting, as well as for coding diagnoses and procedures for reimbursement.

The HIM professional may contribute to quality management by analyzing clinical data that can then be used to monitor performance improvement. The professional may also assist in monitoring resources through utilization management. Risk management, which is designed to reduce risk and liability, and the credentialing process, which ensures that only qualified practitioners can practice in their area of expertise, are two additional departments that the HIM professional may work closely with.

The HIM professional works with other departments in the provision of administrative and research statistics. For example, administration may want to know what the occupancy rate of the facility was for last month. A large teaching hospital may have the professional working with the medical staff to gather data and compile statistics regarding a clinical trial. Health care professionals realize that quality information is a significant part of providing quality care. The HIM professional must work with the medical staff and other interdisciplinary professionals to provide this information.

Financial and Information Systems Management

The HIM professional plays a key role in the financial and information systems in organizations. Systems such as diagnosis related groups (DRGs), resource utilization groups, or ambulatory payment classifications (APCs) mandate that the coding be accurate.

The job of the HIM professional in clinical data management has become highly technical because of the following factors:

- The large number of diagnoses and procedures that need to be coded
- The large number of third-party and review organizations requesting coded data
- Delays in billing and reimbursement if the coding is not accurate

Administration focuses on costs and financial feasibility while striving to provide quality care and services to all patients. Therefore, the HIM professional and CFO must work closely in the handling of budgets, cash flow, coding, sequencing, and reimbursement issues.

Integrated clinical and financial information systems represent another financial management area in which the HIM department plays a key role. The coded data produced by the HIM department are integrated with financial data to provide the administration with the information necessary to make important decisions about quality and profitability. The databases created with the merger of the clinical and financial data are used for reports, statistics, and research.

CONCLUSION

The health record, whether documented on hard copy or through electronic means, is a vital component in the provision of quality care. Current trends in the health care industry, such as providing services across a continuum of care and the development of longitudinal records, make the managing of health information a critical component in the delivery of these services. This information is used by various health care professionals in providing treatment, and the data abstracted from the record can be used for research, reimbursement, and quality management review.

The HIM professional plays an important role in the provision of quality care through providing quality information. The professional should ensure that the data are accurate, timely, and complete. The HIM professional works collaboratively with other members of the interdisciplinary team in sharing responsibility for the creation, maintenance, and protection of this health information.

REFERENCES

1. http://www.ahima.org/about/main.htm
2. E. Huffman, *Health Information Management,* 10th ed. (Berwyn, Ill.: Physicians' Record Company, 1994): 367.
3. http://www.ahima.org/about/main.htm
4. http://www.ahima.org/careers/main.html
5. AHIMA, "Vision 2006: A Framework for the Future" (Chicago: House of Delegates, 1996).
6. http://www.ahima.org/journal/pb/99.10.html

BIBLIOGRAPHY

Abdelhak, M., ed., *Health Information: Management of a Strategic Resource,* 2nd ed. (Philadelphia: W.B. Saunders, 2001).

AHIMA, *Evolving HIM Careers* (Chicago: AHIMA, 1999).

Glondys, B. *Documentation Requirements for the Acute Care Patient Record* (Chicago: AHIMA, 1999).

CHAPTER 2

Content and Structure of the Health Record

Linda S. Kiger

A s noted in Chapter One, a health care facility must demonstrate substantial compliance with the standards of JCAHO in order to be accredited. Included in the Joint Commission standards are benchmarks for the maintenance and adequacy of health records. In addition, federal Conditions of Participation, state departments of health, and other accrediting bodies such as the American Osteopathic Association's Health Facilities Accreditation Program govern health record content. This chapter provides an overview of the major standards that pertain to health record content and describes formats that are typically used to structure health records.

HEALTH RECORD CONTENT

An adequate health record service incorporates all of a patient's pertinent clinical information within a single record. Such consolidation is important for current and continuing care purposes, utilization management, and quality assessment and improvement activities. Based on Joint Commission standards for patient-specific data, the information is used to accomplish the following objectives:

- Facilitate patient care
- Serve as a financial and legal record
- Aid in clinical research
- Support decision analysis
- Guide professional and organizational performance improvement[1]

To ensure thoroughness, all departments that participate in patient care must document their activities in the health record. Thus the specific content of a health record varies with regard to the departments that treat the patient and subsequently record related information. For example, the health record of a patient who receives services from physical and occupational therapy, speech therapy, social service, and dietetics will contain documentation of care from all these departments. The health record of a patient who undergoes surgery may contain records from the surgery department, anesthesiology, and pathology, depending on the services received.

Use of Abbreviations in the Health Record

To maintain the clarity that is so essential to health records, the health care facility should maintain a listing of the abbreviations and symbols that the medical staff has approved for use in documentation. Each abbreviation and symbol should have only one meaning. Diagnoses and procedures should be documented using accepted disease and operative terminology that includes topography and etiology, as appropriate. When information is recorded using unique or numerous abbreviations and symbols, a legend should be included on the forms. The HIM professional is responsible for ensuring that abbreviations are used in health records only when appropriate and that abbreviations do not threaten the objective description of facts essential to both good medical practice and scientific progress.

Joint Commission and State Content Standards

The Joint Commission specifically requires information in the medical record that identifies the patient, supports the diagnosis, justifies the treatment, documents the course of action and subsequent results, and facilitates the continuity of care. Accreditation standards are revised and published quarterly in the Joint Commission's *Accreditation Manual for Hospitals*.[2] The HIM professional should remain abreast of the standards and scoring guides related to the management of health information contained in the latest edition of the manual and in other relevant Joint Commission publications such as the accreditation manuals for ambulatory care and long-term care.[3]

In addition to the Joint Commission requirements, a specific state regulation may also govern other information to be included in the record. The individual state licensing authority is an appropriate reference for state laws or regulations. The AHIMA practice brief "Recommended Regulation and Standard Acquisition for Specific Health Care Settings" is also a useful reference.[4]

The sections that follow describe standards for records involving various types of care or departments or facilities. Included are the following items:

- Inpatient records
- "Observation-status" patient records
- Ambulatory care records
- Emergency care records
- Home health records
- Long-term care and rehabilitation records
- Hospice records
- Mental health records
- Records of other departments; managed care and HMO records

Inpatient Records

Records must be maintained for all inpatients, that is, for all patients admitted to the facility. The Joint Commission standards for inpatient health or medical records require that each record include the following information:[5]

- Patient identification data, including the patient's name, address, date of birth, and the name of any legally authorized representative
- The legal status of patients receiving mental health services
- Any emergency care provided to the patient prior to arrival
- The record and findings of the patient's assessment
- Conclusions or impressions drawn from the medical history and physical examination
- The diagnosis or diagnostic impression
- The reasons for admission or treatment
- The goals of treatment and the treatment plan
- Evidence of known advance directives
- Evidence of informed consent, when required by health care facility policy
- Any diagnostic and therapeutic orders
- All diagnostic and therapeutic procedures and test results
- Test results relevant to the management of the patient's condition
- All operative and other invasive procedures performed, using acceptable disease and operative terminology that includes etiology, as appropriate
- Progress notes made by the medical staff and other authorized individuals
- All reassessments and any revision of the treatment plan
- Clinical observations
- The patient's response to care
- Consultation reports
- Every medication ordered or prescribed for an inpatient
- Every medication dispensed to an inpatient on discharge
- Every dose of medication administered and any adverse drug reaction

- All relevant diagnoses established during the course of care
- Any referrals and communications made to external or internal care providers and to community agencies
- Conclusions at the termination of hospitalization
- Discharge instructions to the patient and family
- Clinical résumés and discharge summaries or a final progress note or transfer summary

The AHIMA practice brief "Documentation Requirements for the Acute Care Inpatient Record" is an additional reference.[6]

Note that Joint Commission standards require that the medical record contain evidence of informed consent for procedures and treatment for which health care facility policy requires such consent.[7] The informed consent form is not to be confused with the authorization for treatment form, which is signed at the time of admission. The term *informed consent* implies that the patient has been informed of the procedures or operation to be performed, of the risks involved, and of the possible consequences. To comply with this requirement, a health care facility representative should discuss the benefits of a proposed action with the patient and review risks, alternatives, subsequent procedures to be followed, and the right to refuse treatment. All discussions and review are documented. (The medical staff and the governing board, consistent with legal requirements for appropriate informed consent, develop the policy on informed consent.)

By signing the consent form, the patient or the patient's representative indicates that he or she has been informed, understands the information, and consents to the procedure or treatment. If, for some reason, the informed consent form is not filed with the health record, the health record must indicate that informed consent was obtained for a given procedure or treatment and should describe the location of the informed consent form. If appropriate, surrogate decision makers are identified and so noted in the patient record.

Observation Patient Records

Records must also be maintained for patients who are on "observation status." Observation beds (distinguished from inpatient beds) can be located in a unit designated for patients on observation status—for instance, ambulatory surgery patients who need additional time to recover or patients who need to be observed following outpatient surgery. The observation may last less than twenty-four hours, or it may extend to the following day. Patients may be admitted to or discharged from the facility through the observation unit.

When observation beds are permitted, written policies and procedures address their type of use by patients, the maximum time of their use, the mechanism for providing appropriate surveillance, and the type of health information system to be used. The medical record information is incorporated into the patient's permanent record, and all pertinent documentation is recorded while the patient remains on observation status.

Ambulatory Care Records

Ambulatory care records are typically generated in ambulatory surgery, health clinics, and physicians' offices. The content standards established by the Joint Commission for facility-sponsored, ambulatory care services require the following information:[8]

- Patient identification
- Relevant history of the illness or injury and of physical findings
- Diagnostic and therapeutic orders
- Clinical observations, including the results of treatment
- Reports of procedures and tests and their results
- Diagnosis or impression
- Patient disposition and any pertinent instructions given for follow-up care
- Immunization record

- Allergy history
- Growth charts for pediatric patients
- Referral information to and from agencies
- For patients receiving outpatient care on a continuing basis, a summary list should contain the following information:

Known significant medical diagnoses and conditions

Known significant operative and invasive procedures

Known adverse and allergic drug reactions

Medications known to be prescribed for or used by the patient

Ambulatory care has received much attention in recent years due to changes in the health care delivery system. Maintaining standards for the quality and content of ambulatory care records is often difficult because of the episodic nature of ambulatory care, the fragmentation of care that can result from the presence of specialty clinics, and the rapid pace that is characteristic of outpatient care, which fosters brief entries of information. To maintain standards, ambulatory care systems must be integrated or networked with the health care facility's clinical information system. Integration allows for the exchange of patient data among providers, coding systems on-line to report required data, a mechanism for protecting patient information confidentiality, and statistical data collection and dissemination. In addition, the integrated system ensures that health care professionals involved in a patient's care have available a valid means of communication regarding that person's total health picture.

The HIM professional should assume an active role in the development or modification of the health record system, according to the type of ambulatory care facility. The Uniform Ambulatory Care Data Set, approved by the National Committee on Vital and Health Statistics, identifies a common core of standard data items with accompanying uniform definitions. The items are recommended for inclusion in records of all ambulatory health care. Data items include patient data, provider data, encounter data, diagnostic services, disposition, patient's expected sources of payment, and total charges.[9]

Emergency Care Records

Joint Commission standards and legal considerations dictate that a health or medical record be maintained on every patient who seeks emergency care and, when feasible, that the emergency record be incorporated into the patient's permanent medical record. The Joint Commission's standards for information to be entered into the emergency care record include the following:[10]

- Identification
- Time and means of arrival
- History of present illness or injury
- Physical findings and vital signs
- Emergency care provided to the patient prior to arrival
- Diagnostic and therapeutic orders
- Reports of procedures, tests, and results
- Clinical observations, including the results of treatment
- Diagnostic impression
- Conclusion at the termination of treatment, including final disposition, the patient's condition at discharge, and any instructions given to the patient or family for follow-up care
- Patient leaving against medical advice

An emergency record is typically one page long. A copy of the form may be sent to the patient's personal physician, with the original retained for the health care facility record.

Home Health Records

Standards for facility-sponsored home care programs include the maintenance of accurate records for every patient receiving care through the pro-

Health Information Management

gram. The records maintained for home care patients should be similar to those maintained for inpatients and ambulatory care patients, and professional staff members in the home care program should have access to the inpatient and ambulatory care records of their patients during the development of written patient care plans.

The federal government has developed guidelines for home health records in programs approved for use by Medicare patients. The Conditions of Participation for Medicare-certified home health agencies require compliance with Outcome and Assessment Information Set (OASIS) collection and transmission requirements.

In the home care record, the progress notes should include documentation of signs and symptoms, treatment or services rendered, any medication administered, the patient's reaction to treatment or medication, any change in the patient's condition, and instructions given to the patient or family. To be Medicare-certified, skilled nursing care must be provided along with physical, speech, or occupational therapy, medical social services, or home health aide services.

The HIM department's responsibilities for record services within the home health care program include

- Record security and procedures for the orderly transfer of the health record among inpatient and ambulatory care facilities and home health care service
- Disclosure of health record information to outside parties
- Implementation of any recommended changes in form design
- Coordination of the transfer of records to and from home health care offices

A publication from AHIMA titled *Documentation and Reimbursement for Home Care and Hospice Programs* provides additional information. The publication includes field-tested model record forms and instructions for their use, record documentation and review guidelines that include documentation for Medicare reimbursement, the Uniform Data Set for

Home Care and Hospice, continuous quality improvement guidelines, a chapter on data and information management, model confidentiality policies, and relevant ICD-9-CM coding information.[11]

Long-Term Care and Rehabilitation Records

A long-term care or nursing facility may be located within or outside the medical facility that administers it. Alternatively, a small health care facility may use the swing-bed method, whereby bed designation can be changed from acute care to skilled care and vice versa, depending on the level of care required by each patient.

The term *nursing home* is typically used to refer to all three levels of long-term care: (1) skilled care, (2) intermediate care, and (3) residential care. Skilled care, the most comprehensive level of care at a nursing facility, is reserved for patients who require skilled nursing care twenty-four hours a day and, on a regular basis, various support services such as medications, injections, and catheterizations. In an intermediate-level facility, the care is not as complex, and the residents require fewer services. At the residential care level, residents' needs may be classified as "assisted living" or as "independent living."

The content of the health record in the nursing facility is similar to that of a health care facility health record, regardless of the level of care provided. Therefore, the same health record forms can be used for both acute and skilled care. However, entries must be made on the front sheet and in the body of the record to identify clearly the date of transfer to and from acute care and skilled care levels. For statistical and financial purposes, the health record must differentiate between the two levels of care. When the patient is transferred from the acute care level to skilled care, a written summary of the acute care stay should be included. The instructions and orders for skilled care should then be entered into the health record as the patient's care continues.

If the nursing facility is located some distance from the health care facility, it may not be feasible, practical, or desirable to transfer the patient's entire health record when the patient is transferred from acute care to

Health Information Management

skilled care. In this case, a clinical résumé is prepared along with nursing care instructions and copies of any pertinent portions of the health record for inclusion in the nursing facility's health record. Additional information on standards for health record services in long-term care facilities is offered in the latest edition of the Joint Commission's *Accreditation Manual for Long Term Care*[12] and AHIMA's *LTC Health Information Practice and Documentation Guidelines.*[13]

Rehabilitation facilities train or retrain individuals who have been disabled by disease or injury to attain the highest possible level of functional ability. As discussed in Chapter One, the Joint Commission or the Commission on Accreditation of Rehabilitations Facilities (CARF) may accredit facilities that provide rehabilitative care. CARF requires that a unit record be maintained for each person admitted to a rehabilitation facility. Documentation in the record should be clear, concise, complete, and prompt. General health record documentation requirements and record-keeping practices are applicable. The HIM professional should consult the appropriate Joint Commission and CARF manuals, as well as state regulatory requirements and the Medicare requirements for more detailed information.

Hospice Records

Hospice care is an alternative to hospital-based acute care for terminally ill patients. The health record for hospice care must be compatible with the records of care provided to the terminally ill patient and the needs of the hospice. HIM professionals must be familiar with the hospice services that are covered and reimbursable under Medicare, Medicaid, private pay, third-party payers, community funds, or other sources, as well as state licensing and health-planning requirements. AHIMA's *Documentation and Reimbursement for Home Care and Hospice Programs* (cited earlier) includes model health record forms and instructions for their use, health record documentation guidelines, a recommended minimum data set, confidentiality guidelines, health record system guidelines, and coding guidelines. Frequently used diagnoses and their corresponding ICD-9-CM codes are also listed.[14]

Mental Health Records

All facilities that provide psychiatric care and that are licensed as hospitals are surveyed under the *Joint Commission's Accreditation Manual for Hospitals.*[15] Facilities that provide psychiatric care but that are not licensed as hospitals are surveyed under the Joint Commission's *Accreditation Manual for Behavioral Health Care.*[16] Such facilities include freestanding alcohol and drug abuse rehabilitation programs and community mental health centers.

In addition to the standard documentation of health records in other settings, mental health records require evaluation and treatment plan entries, flow charting, and psychiatric evaluations. The HIM professional employed in this setting should be familiar with federal and Joint Commission requirements that are applicable throughout the country, as well as with varying state and local regulations. Legal issues and confidentiality concerns are of extreme importance in mental health records. The HIM professional must keep pace with the continual changes in regulations and systems in health information to maintain the most functional clinical information system in the area of mental health.

Records for Other Types of Care

Along with the various types of health records that must be maintained outside acute care facilities, health records are also maintained within the medical facility in other departments and by contracted service organizations. The HIM professional must be familiar with all current managed care contracts and their related record requirements. Departments such as social service or physical therapy also maintain specific health records that may affect the operations of the HIM department.

Many health care facilities have contractual arrangements with HMOs or preferred provider organizations (PPOs) to provide inpatient, emergency, and diagnostic services as requested and authorized by the HMO or PPO. The American Hospital Association (AHA) defines an HMO as "a health care organization that acts as both insurer and provider of comprehensive but specified medical services in return for prospective per capita (capitation) payments."[17] HMOs are financed through fixed premiums paid by members in return for the availability of all services included under the plan. In contrast to a fixed-premium arrangement, PPOs use a fee-for-service system. The PPO panel contracts with providers to offer care to PPO subscribers at a negotiated discounted cost.

In both systems, record-keeping responsibilities must be shared by the organization and the medical facility that provides health record and information services. Written policies should detail the exchange of medical information necessary for acute and continuing patient care and outline procedures for the disclosure of health record information to the patient or an outside party.

Within the health care facility itself, departments other than HIM maintain other types of records to permit continuity of therapy or departmental case studies and reports. During the patient's stay, the daily records of physical therapy, occupational therapy, or social services are maintained more easily in those departments, provided that timely progress notes are entered into the patient's health record. Evaluation and treatment information is incorporated into the health record when treatment or therapy has been completed, either by providing a summary or by inserting the actual documents. The original documents are placed in the permanent health record, and a copy is maintained in the department. Department work sheets designed for temporary use are destroyed after the summary information is recorded in the permanent health record. Work sheets containing notes that could be misinterpreted later should not be a part of the permanent record.

STRUCTURE OF THE HEALTH RECORD

Neither the Joint Commission nor the AHA recommends any specific format or forms for use in medical facility health records. In current practice, however, the health record is typically structured in one of three ways: (1) as a source-oriented record, (2) as a record with integrated progress notes, or (3) as a problem-oriented medical (or health) record.

Source-Oriented Health Record

The traditional medical facility health record is arranged chronologically and structured around the information provider (the medical staff or other health professionals). Thus the health record is divided into sections that indicate the source of documented data. Typical sections may include physicians' notes, clinical laboratory and radiological reports, social service notes, nurses' notes and charts, and so forth. Within each section, information is entered in chronological order. (After discharge, information may be arranged in reverse chronological order to streamline discharge analysis procedures by facilitating the record completion process.) The physician using progress notes, which provide an assessment of existing problems, reasons for therapeutic decisions, and a description of the patient's course of illness during his or her stay, integrates data from the various sources.

Critics of the source-oriented health record cite its lack of consistent organization. Pertinent information may be difficult to find because the record is bulky and does not contain an index to specific items. When properly maintained, however, the source-oriented health record reflects the physician's direction of patient care, his or her communication with others involved in the care of the patient, the course of the patient's illness, and the physician's conclusions.

Records with Integrated Progress Notes

The integrated (or universal) progress notes format enables physicians and other health care professionals to enter all progress notes in chronological order on one form. The chronological recording of progress notes pools data from various disciplines, thereby stimulating improved patient care through shared knowledge.

Advantages and Disadvantages of Integrated Progress Notes

The integrated progress notes system can offer several advantages. Because all notes are concentrated on one form, each professional who shares responsibility for the care of a patient can quickly determine the patient's progress. Equally important, the system promotes the team concept among health professionals and reduces the likelihood that one team member will inadvertently overlook another's documentation or that an unwarranted destruction of significant observations made by the nursing staff will occur. Finally, the system encourages concise and prompt recording of all information (to maintain chronological sequencing) and streamlines the record by reducing the number of specialized forms.

A disadvantage of the integrated progress notes system is that only one individual can document or review progress notes in a health record at any given time. In addition, it may be difficult to identify the professional discipline of recorders unless they sign their notes in full and identify their titles or departments. It also is necessary for the attending physician to differentiate his or her documentation from that of others. Differentiation can be accomplished by having the physician begin his or her notes at the left margin of the form and having all other recorders indent their notes, or vice versa. A final drawback is that progress notes may occasionally appear to conflict when they are documented in proximity and represent the opinions of many health care professionals. For example, because nursing notes often relate to more than therapy, they may seem to contradict notes related solely to therapy.

Conversion to Integrated Progress Notes

Health care facilities that currently do not use the integrated progress notes system but wish to do so must plan the conversion carefully. The appointment of a planning committee that consists of representatives from the HIM department and from each contributing discipline can do much to facilitate the conversion.

The planning committee's role should cover the following functions:

- Outline the reasons for the conversion to the integrated system and list the advantages and disadvantages of the change.
- Develop a form for use in the integrated system.

- Identify the forms that will be superseded by the new one, such as those for physicians' progress notes, nursing notes, respiratory therapy notes, and physical therapy progress notes. (Medication and treatment records, as well as graphic sheets, may still be kept separate from the universal progress notes.)

- Develop guidelines that describe the kinds of notes to be included in the integrated system, assign authority to write them, identify the individuals who are to make entries, stipulate the locations wherein they may enter data, and control accessibility to the records.

- Develop plans for the initial orientation of staff members involved in the changeover and for the subsequent orientation of new employees.

- Obtain final approval from the medical record committee, the medical staff, and the administration.

Without the strong support of these groups, the system may be difficult to implement.

Problem-Oriented Medical Records

In the problem-oriented medical record (POMR) system, clinical information is organized by dividing the record into four sections—database, problem list, initial plan, and progress notes—and recording the information according to specific patient problems. First introduced by a physician, Lawrence Weed, in the 1960s, the POMR system represents a unique approach to the practice of medicine and to the recording of medical information. Structured to provide a total approach to patient care, the POMR enumerates the patient's problems; progress notes, orders, and all other documentation are referenced to the particular problems that they concern. All the documentation in the health record centers on the patient's individual problems and on the steps necessary to solve those problems. Because this method allows all of the patient's problems—medical and otherwise—to be brought into relationship with one another, it avoids the fragmentation that often results when the source-oriented approach to documentation is used. The POMR may therefore help physicians treat patients more effectively.

Health Information Management

The Database

The initial component of the POMR is its database—the documentation of the patient's expression of his or her problems in his or her own words. The database includes information on the present illness, the patient's history, the review of body systems, the patient's family and social history, and the physical examination. This information is included in all records and used by all members of the health care team in the diagnosis and treatment of the patient.

The Problem List

The second component of the POMR—the problem list—is an enumeration of all the patient's problems, whether they are medical, family-related, work-related, or social. Nonmedical problems are given greater attention in the POMR than in other kinds of health records, thereby reflecting the importance of their impact on the patient's health. For example, the root cause of a psychiatric patient's depression might be a problem within his or her family. The patient's list of problems is developed by the physician from the database, and each problem is numbered, titled, and dated. If the problem is resolved later, that fact is noted and dated in the record. With this type of medical record, care must be taken to ensure that a condition that is either suspected or ruled out appears as a component of a treatment plan and not as a problem.

The Initial Plan

The third component of the POMR is the initial plan. In this section of the health record, the physician outlines a plan for collecting further information and for diagnostic or therapeutic treatment. To ensure that the plan clearly correlates with the problems, each part of it is numbered to correspond to the problem that it seeks to address.

The Progress Notes

The fourth component of the POMR—the progress notes—documents the patient's progress relative to the physician's goals. Progress notes are written in the subjective-objective-assessment-plan (SOAP) format.

The subjective statement includes the symptomatic complaints the patient voices that cannot necessarily be measured or strictly defined. The objective statements are measurable, observable findings, such as blood pressure, respiration rate, pulse rate, and laboratory test results. The assessment is a statement of what is currently happening with the patient; it may indicate the present condition of the patient and any changes in his or her condition. Finally, the plan indicates the physician's course of action for the patient, including steps that must be taken immediately or in the future as part of the long-term plan.

Advantages and Disadvantages of the Problem-Oriented Health Record

A major advantage of the POMR is its holistic approach to patient care. The POMR format makes it easy for each member of the health care team to follow a patient's course of treatment, understand the method of treatment, and recognize the problem for which a particular medication or test was ordered. Thus the health care team can better understand the patient's problems, see their interrelationship, and decide the best way to proceed with treatment. In short, the POMR can be an important information link among all individuals directly involved with the patient's care. The record can be initiated at the ambulatory care level and carried through inpatient care without fragmentation. This feature may be especially useful for teaching hospitals, where many individuals make documentation in the record.

Moreover, the POMR can facilitate self-assessments and other quality assessment activities because of its logical, organized format. Equally important, the standardized organization of information is compatible with the computer-based patient record (CPR). Although the POMR has not been widely used in the past, it is finding new popularity for this reason.

A disadvantage of the POMR format is the time and commitment needed to transition to such a system. Implementation of the POMR, or any portion of it, requires the support of the medical staff, the administration, and HIM professionals. Although one or more clinical services may elect to adopt the POMR approach, reluctance on the part of individuals to change their recording patterns sometimes makes it difficult to obtain acceptance of the POMR system from the entire medical staff. In addition, training must be provided to educate those who work with the system. The costs of in-service training for the POMR system would be similar to those necessitated by any change in documentation activities.

A facility unwilling to change the entire record format to the POMR system may elect to use the SOAP format for the progress notes and use the integrated progress note format. Many medical schools encourage the use of the SOAP note format as a good communication tool among the medical student, intern, resident, and attending physician, because each of these individuals has access to the opinions of others on the case and can make decisions accordingly.

Records of Discharged Patients

The records of discharged patients can be assembled in a variety of ways, regardless of the method used for record documentation. The Joint Commission does not mandate a specified format nor require a reordering of the chart information at discharge. Therefore, the medical facility can make its decision based on its own needs for referral to the health record information in the future.

Health record textbooks such as *HIM Technology. An Applied Approach* by Merida Johns[18] and *Health Information: Management of a Strategic Resource* by Mervat Abdelhak[19] describe a universal chart order or patient record content structure that may be adapted and modified by the health care facility. Although the list is certainly not all-inclusive, it does provide guidance in creating a chart order specific to the needs of the facility.

To save time, some HIM departments have eliminated the assembly or reordering process of the record at discharge. Instead, coders use an unassembled record, and the record is filed in the permanent file.

UNIT RECORD SYSTEM

The unit record is a type of health record that combines, in a single record, all the information relative to the medical care that an individual receives during stays in the health care facility, during visits to the ambulatory care departments, the emergency department, or other facilities, and for treatments in a sponsored home care program. The unit record is maintained to provide members of the health care facility and medical staff with information on the patient's current and past conditions, procedures that have been performed, and responses to therapy. As such, the unit record cannot remain in the domain of any one staff member or patient care area. The HIM department must exercise authority in retrieving the record from any location for purposes of patient care. At times, it may be necessary for the CEO or medical staff chairperson to support the HIM department director in enforcing procedures for authorized users to gain access to the health record.

Content of the Unit Record

The Joint Commission does not specifically require that a health care facility maintain a unit record; however, it does require that all relevant inpatient, ambulatory care, emergency, urgent, or immediate care records be assembled when a patient receives care. The intent of these information management standards is to promote continuity of care, both over time and among providers. If more than one clinic in the health care facility keeps a record of the patient, each record must note that there is additional information elsewhere.[20]

When feasible, the unit record includes documentation of home care sponsored by health care facilities. For these sponsored home care patients, the unit record is held in the home care office for timely updated and reference, but it must be readily accessible for use in clinic or emergency department visits and admissions to the health care facility. Inpatient stays followed by continuing care in the institution's ambulatory care facility or home care program can present problems in completing records, filing loose reports, and coding and abstracting. A patient who is

Health Information Management

discharged to the long-term care unit or hospice unit also must have a record maintained for that stay. Linkage to the health care facility's record information is important, but a unit record in this instance may be impossible to maintain.

In addition, reports prepared by any outside services such as pathology services or clinical therapy tests are filed as part of the patient's health record. When the health care facility contracts for outside professional services in areas such as physical therapy, the report of service provided and the patient's progress is entered into his or her individual health record at the facility. When physician services are contracted for emergency care, the original report of findings, care provided, and disposition of the patient are filed in the health record. The emergency department physician is also entitled to a copy of that department's record.

Arrangement of Information in the Unit Record

Information in the unit record may be arranged in chronological or reverse-chronological order. In chronological records, patient care information is arranged in the order that events and findings occur. Recall that *chronological order* refers both to a single episode of care and to multiple episodes of inpatient or outpatient care. Thus after an inpatient has been discharged, the individual record sheets pertaining to his or her stay will be assembled in chronological order for physician entries, diagnostic reports, and nursing entries, along with visits to the ambulatory care or emergency departments and any visits of staff members providing home care to the patient.

When a patient has had more than one episode of care as an inpatient or outpatient, a record is maintained by incorporating and arranging visits in reverse-chronological order, with the most recent visit on top. However, the information within each visit remains in chronological order.

Health care facilities may also choose to organize the information within each episode in reverse-chronological fashion. In this case, the most recent episode of care or note is positioned at the top of each section. If neither of these options is used, analysts checking the health record for completeness simply include all papers or data in a given section of the record. Although this speeds up the assembly process, it impedes quick data retrieval.

Benefits of the Unit Record System

The value of the unit record for patient care and study purposes must be weighed against the extra costs of the time and equipment needed to track its location at all times and to retrieve and dispatch records as needed. In addition, everyone involved in the use of the unit record must be sensitive to the need to make the record readily accessible at all times. Many in health care believe that the savings that result from the elimination of or reduction in duplicate patient care records that are maintained in various clinical and therapeutic departments offset these drawbacks. Quality patient care is also enhanced by a record that facilitates retrieval of all information about a specific patient in one location.

Format of the Unit Record

Members of the medical and administrative staff involved in the medical record review function are also responsible for standardizing the format of the medical record, including its arrangement and form design. Usually, the arrangement of the record maintained on the nursing unit is quite different from that of the record prepared for permanent filing. The standardized arrangement facilitates making entries, referencing material, reviewing the record for completeness, assessing the quality of care provided, and abstracting for reporting and collecting statistical data.

The type of folder used to house the health record provides options such as the placement of inpatient information on one side of the folder and all other information on the other side. Dividers in the record also separate less frequently addressed information from key components such as the history and physical examination or the clinical résumé.

The unit record for a patient with multiple admissions or a long period of ambulatory care often requires more than one folder. When multiple volumes are needed for a particular patient's record, it is important to number the folders and to identify the total number of folders that are issued. For example, when a unit record requires three folders, the folders are identified as volume 1 of 3, volume 2 of 3, and volume 3 of 3. Innovations and systems that simplify the recording, review, or timely retrieval of information are encouraged, and these systems should maintain quality and basic record content requirements.

ALTERNATIVES TO THE UNIT RECORD SYSTEM

Health care institutions with affiliated ambulatory care facilities may find the unit record system unworkable. When it is not feasible to combine all documentation into a single record of inpatient care, ambulatory care, emergency care, home care, hospice care, and long-term care, a cross-referencing system can be used to identify the patient and integrate his or her component health records. This may be useful with distant satellite clinics or long-term care facilities that preclude the combination of all information into a unit record. It is particularly important that there be a process for ensuring the ready retrieval and availability of a patient's component health records when that person is admitted to the central health care facility or appears for an ambulatory care appointment at a satellite center. A record location or tracking system should be implemented. It may be a stand-alone personal computer system or an interface with the facility's mainframe information system.

Such systems, which typically use bar codes for input, provide timely information about the location of a record and some historical information about its past movement. These systems are also used to generate sign-out slips for "outguides" and to provide a method for generating a pull list when records are requested. An outguide file folder in a manual system is used to replace a record that has been removed from the permanent file location. The outguide stays in the file until the record is replaced. Among other benefits over a manual outguide system, computerized systems improve record access, and facilitate record retrieval. They also generate various reports on record activity and staff workload, which are useful to the department director in productivity studies, staffing decisions, and quality assessment and control. A chart-tracking system should provide the ability to process an inquiry of chart location by medical record number, check a record in and out by location and requestor, and display the status of any record.

When a computerized system is not available, a manual procedure can be devised to incorporate copies of inpatient discharge summaries and diagnostic tests into ambulatory care, home care, hospice care, and long-term care records. The inpatient record should also include summarized data from other records. The goal is that summary or transfer data will be available in the event of a scheduled admission to the health care facility. It is important to establish systems for maintaining and providing the health record information as needed to authorized individuals. All clinical information relevant to a patient should be readily available to the health care providers.

Health care facilities serving a transient population, such as facilities in a resort area, often have no need to maintain a unit record system. However, for the more permanent population that such facilities service, a single record system should be maintained for all inpatient admissions.

CONCLUSION

Effective information management plays a crucial role in a successful health care facility operation. Whatever health record system is developed and maintained by a health care facility, the HIM professional has significant responsibility in its operation. Whether computer-based or paper-based, the health record must be complete, accurate, and available to authorized individuals.

The *2002 Comprehensive Accreditation Manual for Hospitals* focuses on effective organizationwide information management.[21] The standards are organized around the functions most relevant to patient care rather than around the hospital's departments, services, and professional disciplines. Hence, the chapters from past editions that dealt with medical record services, quality assessment and improvement, and utilization review were eliminated from this text in favor of chapters on information management, organizational performance improvement, and patient assessment. These changes affect the HIM professional's ability to maintain the health record of the facility and to prepare for and participate in the Joint Commission survey process.

REFERENCES

1. Joint Commission on Accreditation of Healthcare Organizations, *2002 Comprehensive Accreditation Manual for Hospitals* (Oakbrook Terrace, Ill.: Joint Commission, 2001).
2. Ibid.
3. Joint Commission on Accreditation of Healthcare Organizations, *2002-2003 Comprehensive Accreditation Manual for Long Term Care* (Oakbrook Terrace, Ill.: Joint Commission, 2001); Joint Commission, *2002–2003 Comprehensive Accreditation Manual for Ambulatory Health Care* (Oakbrook Terrace, Ill.: Joint Commission, 2001).
4. AHIMA, Practice Brief, "Practice Guidelines for Managing Health Information," *Journal of AHIMA* 69, no. 4 (April 1998).
5. Joint Commission, *2002 Comprehensive Accreditation Manual for Hospitals*.
6. AHIMA, Practice Brief, "Practice Guidelines for Managing Health Information," *Journal of AHIMA* 72, no. 3 (March 2001).
7. Joint Commission, *2002 Comprehensive Accreditation Manual for Hospitals*.
8. Ibid.
9. U.S. Department of Health and Human Services, "The Uniform Ambulatory Care Data Set," in *Report of the National Committee on Vital and Health Statistics and Its Interagency Task Force in the Uniform Ambulatory Care Data Set* (Washington, D.C.: DHHS, 1989).
10. Joint Commission, *2002 Comprehensive Accreditation Manual for Hospitals*.
11. AHIMA, *Documentation and Reimbursement for Home Care and Hospice Programs* (Chicago: AHIMA, 2001).
12. Joint Commission, *2002–2003 Comprehensive Accreditation Manual for Long Term Care*.
13. AHIMA, *LTC Health Information Practice and Documentation Guidelines* (Chicago: AHIMA, 2001).
14. AHIMA, *Documentation and Reimbursement for Home Care and Hospice Programs* (Chicago: AHIMA, 2001).
15. Joint Commission, *2002 Comprehensive Accreditation Manual for Hospitals*.

16. Joint Commission on Accreditation of Healthcare Organizations, *2001–2002 Comprehensive Accreditation Manual for Behavioral Healthcare* (Oakbrook Terrace, Ill.: Joint Commission, 2001).
17. American Hospital Association, *Hospital Statistics* (Chicago: AHA, 2001).
18. M. Johns, et al., *HIM Technology: An Applied Approach* (Chicago: AHIMA, 2002).
19. M. Abdelhak, ed., *Health Information: Management of a Strategic Resource,* 2nd ed. (Philadelphia: W.B. Saunders, 2001).
20. Joint Commission, *2002 Comprehensive Accreditation Manual for Hospitals.*
21. Joint Commission, *2002 Comprehensive Accreditation Manual for Hospitals.*

WEB SITES

www.ahima.org

www.aha.org

www.jcaho.org

Health Information Management

CHAPTER 3

The Emergence of Electronic Patient Record Systems

Desla R. Mancilla

utomated health information systems are referred to by a variety of names: computerized patient records (CPR), electronic patient records (EPR), even electronic record systems (ERS). In essence, each of these acronyms describes a complex and integrated electronic system that is used to collect, store, and manage health information.

For centuries, health records were kept in paper form or were not kept at all. With the advent of the technological revolution and the increasing mobility of the world's population, the need for more sophisticated record-keeping systems has emerged. Health records are no longer used simply to recall the health care history of an individual; they are now the crux of elaborate health information networks. Health records are now used in aggregate form for everything from developing public health policy to serving as the basis for Medicare program budgeting.

System vendors are inundating the marketplace with a wide variety of electronic record management solutions. Systems for the creation of on-line records, optical storage programs for storing traditional paper-based health records, and Internet-based information access systems are just a few of the technologies available for managing health information access and use. However, a single system for the automation of every aspect of health record management is not yet a reality in the health care arena. It is important to understand how the computerization of individual health information over the past twenty-five years has led to the increasingly complex and integrated mix of systems we now call *electronic patient record systems.* Without these intermediate steps of automating practical health information functions, the reality of total computerized patient record systems could not be realized. The evolution of these basic functions is described in the sections to follow.

Master Patient Index

One of the most basic functions performed in a health information department is the operation of a master patient index (MPI). Automation of the MPI function appeared in the early 1980s and offered an efficient solution to the unwieldy and time-consuming process of manually alphabetizing and filing cards that included patient name, record number, and visit details. With the development of integrated delivery networks composed of some combination of acute care facilities, long-term care organizations, primary care providers, facility-based fitness programs, and other customer care settings, the need for a cross-facility MPI has all but demanded the computerization of this function.

Chart Tracking

The demand for information within a single facility is tremendous. It is even more apparent within a multiple provider care setting. Although electronic access to the entire patient record is becoming more prominent in the industry, a significant number of facilities still maintain paper health records. For these facilities, computerized chart tracking is essential in order to efficiently locate and route records as needed. Combined with bar coding that reduces manual entry into the computer system, automated chart tracking is the most efficient and accurate method of managing health record storage and retrieval.

Health Information Management

Abstracting

Abstracting is another traditional health information function that has been greatly improved in terms of both efficiency and quality due to automation of the process. Prior to the automation of this function, coders or abstractors collected up to one hundred unique data elements and manually completed abstract forms. The forms were then tabulated, aggregated, and summarized. Electronic abstracting has allowed for the dynamic reporting of collected data elements.

Cancer Registry

Automation of cancer registry functions such as abstracting, accession registration, and follow-up have promoted the collection and reporting of cancer data. With the development of electronic communication methodologies, both state and national cancer databases receive data in a timely fashion. And, even more important, once the data are available electronically, the opportunities for data analysis are endless. The trending of data to determine cancer introduction and spread is now an efficient process resulting in public policies that are designed to combat cancer throughout the country.

Vital Statistics

Birth and death recording that was performed manually prior to the 1980s was often inaccurate and untimely. Computer programs that are used to collect and disseminate vital statistics data are now commonplace and frequently mandated by state departments of health.

Record Completion

The first generation of record completion systems were rudimentary programs allowing for the assignment of record deficiencies to a responsible party. Subsequent reporting capabilities allowed lists to be printed by responsible parties; records could be pulled for completion when the responsible party arrived in the health information department to complete his or her records. Later, reporting by individual physician data allowed for the development of a "no bed list" and other programs to record delinquency and enforcement. Emerging record completion systems often have an Internet-based access component that allows for the completion of records from the physician's office or other locations.

Coding

Coding, which has long been acknowledged as the bread and butter of the HIM profession, has benefited immensely from the automation of the process. Along with systems that allow the HIM professional to quickly navigate to the appropriate codes in an electronic environment (a significant benefit in itself), there are systems that include links to on-line references regarding acceptable code application for specific billing circumstances. In addition, the use of automated DRG-grouping programs allowed facilities to efficiently monitor their inpatient billing processes. Automated systems that group codes into ambulatory payment classifications (APCs) provide this same benefit in outpatient care settings.

Transcription

Not only can programs be used for typing or transcribing medical reports but there are programs for digitally recording the voice of the individual dictating the reports. The time-consuming revisions necessitated by a manual system were long ago replaced by computerized systems for report creation and revision. Some systems are making use of voice recognition technology, that is, the computer program performs the transcription of the recording. However, this technology has not yet been proven stable in the typical transcription production environment.

With the growing dependence on automation of these individual functions, total electronic patient record systems are imminent.

TYPES OF AUTOMATED SYSTEMS

The long-sought-after goal of health record automation is the achievement of a totally paperless health information environment. In order to achieve this goal, both the creation of the information and its ultimate storage mechanism must be electronic and paperless. Today's technologies support this goal, yet there are very few, if any, truly paperless health information systems.

Paperless Electronic Patient Record Systems

Looking first at the automation of health information from the perspective of the patient caregiver, the systems necessary to facilitate a paperless environment must support the ease of data collection and access.

The analysis of documentation practices within a hospital emergency department can clearly depict how clinical and information systems can be integrated to meet the needs of the user. From the moment a patient enters the door (and even before in the case of patients arriving via ambulance) until the time of patient discharge or transfer, the patient care process demands the immediate availability of data for treating the patient.

Emergency departments are traditionally fast-paced, and the staff often performs triage assessment even before the patient is registered in the system. The triage process is used to assess the significance of the patient's condition and to stage the individual for treatment, based on the collective need of the patient population currently being seen in the facility. Once this assessment is performed, the patient is registered in the hospital information system, where the collection of demographic and billing information is initiated. After the patient is in an emergency department bed, there is a need for patient flow tracking, as ancillary testing is often not performed in the emergency department itself. Instead, patients are often moved from one area to another within the facility and, depending on the length of time they are gone, other patients can be treated in the emergency department during their absence. Entire systems have surfaced to manage this process within emergency departments. Another consideration is the need for access to the patient's past health information, which is often accomplished through searching another computer system for previous visit detail.

Some clinical information systems have both a clinical component and an information component. For example, EKG systems today are computer systems that collect and analyze the patient's physical signs. Human care providers then often interpret the results of the test. It is important to note, however, that this is not always necessary, as many clinical systems use expert system, artificial intelligence, or knowledge-based technology, with rules replicating the steps that human care providers go through in interpreting disease processes. In essence, many of these clinical systems can both collect and analyze, or diagnose, the physical condition of the patient. However, the general acceptance of computer diagnosis without human review is weak.

Taking this scenario a step further, perhaps the results of the EKG indicate the need for respiratory therapy. A therapist presents to the patient's bedside, provides treatment, and enters the information necessary to create documentation in the electronic respiratory system. The clinical values are interpreted by the computer system, producing alerts and confirmations so the therapist can ensure that appropriate treatment protocols are followed. All the while, the nursing staff is performing their assessment of the patient. Elements like temperature, pulse, and respirations, communications with the patient to determine pain levels, and recording of the responses and actions are being documented at the bedside to create the legal medical record. These nursing care systems, often referred to as bedside care systems, promote the efficient collection of patient information through a variety of input mechanisms. Generally, these bedside documentation programs allow the user to select from a preprogrammed list of common patient responses in order to speed the entry process. Patient identification is often confirmed in the system by having the care provider "swipe" a bar-coded wristband. These efficiencies reduce the need to key in patient information, which is a highly resource-intensive process. In fact, one of the major obstacles that must be overcome in order to achieve caregiver acceptance of systems of this type is their perceived inconvenience.

Health Information Management

There are even automated pharmaceutical dispensing systems that fall under the wide umbrella known as *clinical information equipment*. Systems like these allow the user to enter a code representing a specific medication. The most common dosages and forms of these drugs are then dispensed in vending machine style. The data collected in this system regarding the medication dosage and frequency are then passed to the electronic patient record system where they are ultimately available for storage and retrieval. Systems of these types reduce the laborious and time-consuming process of transporting drugs from the pharmacy to the desired location. In emergency situations, immediate delivery of medication that is available through dispensing systems such as those described can significantly improve the patient care process.

How do the systems referred to in this section support the development of an EPR system? Through complex integration mechanisms, the output (progeny) of each system is captured electronically and then sent to a final destination. That final destination is the EPR system. A term sometimes used synonymously, yet erroneously, with EPR is *data repository*. The EPR serves the purpose of creating, storing, and managing individual patient records, whereas a data repository stores elements beyond those available in a traditional health record. For example, a data repository might hold statistical data like patient length-of-stay data (which can be derived from the EPR but are not actually part of the patient record).

The major benefit of a fully automated, paperless system is that the information is immediately available from the point of registration until and after discharge, whenever and wherever it is needed within the organization. This is quite different from paper-based systems that generally become automated later in the treatment process.

Image-Based EPR Systems

If a totally paperless system can be developed, why is there still such emphasis on optical scanning or image-based systems? Quite simply, the complexity of data interchange between multiple systems is, as yet, an insurmountable challenge. Every electronic system has its own proprietary methodologies. Teaching computers to communicate with one another using a common protocol is a daunting task, and purchasing a front-line computer system for every area involved with the patient care process is still too cost-prohibitive for most facilities. However, as technology in health care data collection continues to advance, it is expected that the cost will decrease and the ease of use will increase. Remember the first digital cameras to hit the marketplace? They were extremely expensive and difficult to use; results were often unreliable. Look at them now—affordable and easy to use. That change occurred over a brief period of time. History points to this pattern repeatedly, leading to the conclusion that we can expect similar advances in health information automation.

Optical imaging systems are an intermediate step leading toward a fully automated system. Similar to the discussion previously presented, an optical-imaging-based system is often a complexly integrated process. But by virtue of the fact that there are still many systems in use that create paper output, it is an important step in achieving total automation. Some see optical imaging as a necessary evil. Although the final result is an integrated and automated health record, the process required to achieve that result is very labor-intensive and time-prohibitive. Instead of, or in addition to, capturing output electronically from other systems and then transmitting those data to the EPR, optical imaging systems make use of scanning technology that makes a copy (image) of a paper document. Equate this to a copy machine that makes a copy and stores it in the copier.

The laborious nature of the optical imaging process is due, in part, to the steps needed to prepare the paper documents for the imaging process. Staples must be removed, tears taped, rough spots smoothed, and bent corners unfurled. Failure to take these precautions in the document preparation process results in paper jams and frustration, even with the best scanning equipment available today. The most sophisticated scanning equipment is high-speed and is capable of processing multiple pages at once in a batch scanning process. However, damaged documents often must be handled on an individual basis. In order to ensure that the imaged documents are usable, a quality review process is necessary. In essence, this practice requires human assessment of each image to ensure that it is readable.

In addition, to facilitate the retrieval of stored information an indexing mechanism is required. Indexing is based on some type of identifying information for each unique document. Most often, indexing is accomplished through the use of a bar code that identifies the form type; for example, a bar code that documents the history and physical exam taken by the health care provider is printed on all H&P (history and physical) forms.

In the absence of bar codes (or sometimes in addition to them), optical character recognition (OCR) technology can be used. OCR makes use of a technology that compares a printed title, word, or string of words to a previously stored digital image of the same word or collection of words. If the images match, the system can determine whether the form is an H&P form, a Discharge Summary, or some other form type. The bar code or OCR string, combined with specific patient identifying information (like a patient account or record number), allows the system to quickly locate a specific patient's record and then a specific form within that record.

Most optical-image-based systems combine information that is received both electronically (through, for example, system interfaces) and through scanning. Although the end result of optically scanned health records at first glance seems to be the same as a paperless system, there are some notable differences. The major difference is that in a paperless EPR, all patient information is immediately available from the point of its original inception. In an optical-imaging-based system, parts of the record are originally created in paper form and are later scanned into the system. The logistics of this process are often such that the information is not scanned into the system until after the patient is discharged; thus there can be significant delays in getting the data into the system. In addition, making revisions to scanned documents is an awkward process requiring the overlay of previously processed documents. In a paperless

EPR system, revisions are automatically tracked and monitored through electronic mechanisms.

Finally, retrieval from an optical-imaging-based system is largely a function of the indexing process, whereas a paperless system can allow retrieval through a large variety of other, more discrete sources.

Legacy Systems

The first movement toward health information automation was the introduction of housewide hospital information systems (HIS). Most versions of this product were introduced in the early 1980s and included various software programs to manage a variety of health care functions. Today, HISs are often referred to as legacy systems. Initially, health care billing packages were the mainstay of HISs, followed shortly thereafter by medical record packages for automating the functions discussed earlier in this chapter. Because of the enormous expense of purchasing these housewide HISs, they stayed in place for many years. In fact, many organizations poured money into these massive mainframe systems, even after more efficient personal-computer-based (PC-based) systems were introduced. But many facilities had spent so much money on the purchase of and upgrades to their HISs that they couldn't bring themselves to part with them. It is difficult to weigh the value of a HIS against the value of a collection of PC systems; each serves its own purpose but is integrated to form a comprehensive global information system. The disadvantage of HISs is that they are sold "as is" in a mass sales environment. Many hospitals purchased the exact same product. The base product could be used the same way in every location except that every health care environment has its own unique needs. Therefore, entire information technology (IT) department programming staffs were built to develop modifications to base programs in order to create a more flexible and customized HIS.

Today, legacy systems still play an important role in the developing EPR focus. They often serve to feed basic demographic information that is collected at the registration process to the EPR or other receiving system. Some legacy systems have expanded, over time, to include order entry, test results, pharmacy management, and other modules. In these cases, the information is often still collected by the legacy system and then passed to the EPR as needed.

Stand-Alone and Networked Systems

Completing the mix of technology that works together to create a comprehensive EPR are stand-alone and networked systems. Some very specialized data collection needs are met through stand-alone PCs, like birth certificate or cancer registry systems. For example, information regarding the admission of a newborn child is transmitted from the HIS through an interface or some other transmission protocol to the birth reporting system. Data regarding birth details and neonatal health are collected in the birth certificate system and then passed to the appropriate state agency for processing. Sometimes the data collected in the birth certificate system are ultimately needed in the HIS or EPR. In this case, bidirectional interfaces are used to send data to or receive it from one source or another. The problem with stand-alone systems is that unless the data are transmitted to another system, the information they yield is only available at the specific stand-alone PC that was used to collect them.

To reduce the problem of single-access sites, networked systems developed. In reality, EPR systems are almost exclusively based on network system technology. This technology makes use of the file server concept in which a PC file server stores data until another PC in the network needs them. The requesting PC is known as *the client.* Multiple clients are connected to each file server. And when the term *connected* is used, it does not necessarily mean a physical connection between the server and client. Emerging wireless communication technology, such as "Bluetooth" technology, is making data transfer on demand a reality. Also, radio frequency and other wireless technologies enable the broadcasting of information from one system to another without physical cabling between machines. Although these technologies are fairly new to the marketplace, they represent the future of data interchange. The statement "the devil is in the details" is nowhere more true than in discussions of network system technology. Hardware, software, and communication methodologies all have specific requirements that must work together in concert to achieve the desired result of a seamless EPR system.

Data Collection

The most difficult aspect of automating health information is the development of efficient data entry mechanisms. As a matter of practicality, health care providers will accept no system unless it offers ease of use. The data fields of the feeder systems are generally populated through a variety of mechanisms. For systems that collect information as part of the care provision process, the input mechanism must be some type of hands-free approach, or at least include a "pick list" program capability so that providers can select from a list of standard entries or codes as they are caring for the patient. Of course, these standard entries must allow for customization as needed. Other standard input mechanisms include optical wands to read bar codes that input identifying and medication information. Some systems are now making use of speech-input mechanisms; however, these are not yet widely used or accepted by the physician, nursing, or ancillary staff communities.

Inputting data into the EPR system is largely a matter that is determined by the original source. Paper-based information gets scanned into the system, whereas electronic information reaches the EPR through individual interfaces, an interface engine, or some other source of data transfer such as bi-synchronous communication, a character-oriented data-link-layer protocol,[1] or file transfer protocol (FTP).

An interface engine translates data from the originating system into a standard format that can be accepted by the receiving EPR system. For example, in the originating system the code for a patient's sex might be "F" for female or "M" for male. The EPR might expect the code to be "1" for female or "2" for male. Therefore, the job of the interface engine is to translate the codes from the originating system into the codes that are expected by the EPR or other receiving system.

Health Information Management

System Interrelationships and Integration

When considering data transfer and integration between various systems, two concepts require assessment: (1) the collective group of technical issues known as integration methodologies and (2) the timing of data transfer. When data from numerous systems must reach the EPR, the use of network technology, along with fiber optics, wire cabling, or wireless technology is necessary to create the communication structure between systems.

Data are transferred in one of two modes: (1) real time or (2) batch transfer. *Real-time transfer* refers to the concept that when the data are created in the originating system, they are immediately passed to the receiving system. This type of data transfer is more system-resource-intensive than batch transfers that wait to send grouped data at specific time intervals or at the occurrence of specific events. For example, a "batch send" message may be developed to transfer all of an individual patient's data at discharge, which would be considered a specific event. Another example might be to transfer a collective group of many patients' EKG data from the EKG system to the EPR every fifteen minutes, which would represent a batch transfer based on time intervals.

Data Analysis and System Processing

Once data are in the EPR system, they are used for a multitude of purposes. Those data represent the legal medical record of the patient and, as such, are used to support past and future treatment and justify any issues related to health care. Many systems are developed with workflow processing rules, which make assumptions regarding when certain individuals need to access and use the record. For example, when a record becomes available in the EPR it is needed by the hospital coding staff to apply diagnostic and procedure codes. Once that has happened, the billing department must access portions of the record for inclusion in the claims submission or adjudication process. When a patient is readmitted, the care providers need access to the previous electronic records. In these examples, most EPR workflow processing rules guide how the records are sent to those who need them in order to perform their job functions. In the case of patient readmission, for example, a system rule might be present that automatically routes the previous records to the floor where the patient is currently being treated. Some systems also manage certain workflow functions through the use of age-tracking mechanisms. Like other automated programs, the system tracks how long it takes to complete the coding or the release of information or note the record completion processes. These efficiencies further illustrate the benefits of EPR systems.

Information Output and Reporting

Perhaps the major benefit of EPR systems can be found in their ability to produce data for analysis and decision making in individual-specific, summarized, or aggregate form. Most often this output is in the form of standard or custom reports that can either be displayed and manipulated electronically or printed as paper reports.

In today's health care environment, the variety of decisions made based on aggregate data run the gamut from very simple to extraordinarily complex. Because the EPR replaces the paper-based record, all reports available in a paper environment are also available from the EPR. But the added benefit is that once the information is in electronic form, it can be manipulated to create the output specified by the user. Paper-based reports are often in a standard format; the user gets only the information that has been predefined as needing to appear on that report. Today's health care environment requires a more flexible approach to reporting. Through the use of report-writing software programs, the EPR allows for the development of customized reports by using standardized query languages (SQLs) to extract specific data elements that meet specific criteria for reporting. In addition, every data element is searchable in an EPR, whereas in paper-based systems only those elements that have been abstracted into some automated format can be reported on.

A clarification is necessary here. Even though every element can be searched for in an EPR system, this is not a standard approach. Instead, only indexed elements are generally searched for in the reporting process. Even though every element can be found, it is inefficient to search hundreds or thousands of records for a nonindexed data element.

Reports can be displayed in a variety of output methods. Traditional paper reports are still widely used and distributed within most organizations. However, a computer-based output screen that can be directed to intranet sites allows for broad access within an organization's secured Web environment. Reports can also be developed, stored electronically, and downloaded into other programs for further manipulation or analysis as required.

Health Insurance Portability and Accountability Act

Touted at the time of its inception as being the most sweeping change to the U.S. health care system since the creation of Medicare, the Health Insurance Portability and Accountability Act (HIPAA; see Chapter Two) is refocusing on the need to protect health information from inappropriate access or use. The federal regulations generated by HIPAA continue to support the need for timely access to health information, thereby recognizing that the automation of health information is a good thing. Yet the underlying message sent by HIPAA is that it is irresponsible for the provider to make health care information available in automated form for his or her own convenience, or for the patient's convenience, without the benefit of a sound security structure. Security is the means of maintaining privacy.

Three sections of the HIPAA regulations that fall into the traditional realm of the HIM professional's responsibilities are collectively known as Administrative Simplification. The compliance date for the privacy rule is April 14, 2003. This section of the rule specifies patient access rights and provider compliance in regard to keeping patient information private. The challenge of meeting these demands is more encompassing in an

EPR environment because the initial intent of automating health information was to make the information available quickly and on a wide distribution range. EPR systems do not limit access within the four walls of a single organization. By design, they are meant to distribute information on demand. The vendor community approached the access needs as their first research and development priority. The user community accepted the fact that there were perhaps some security weaknesses and justified this acceptance by acknowledging that they were only sharing information within their own organization. Over time, organizational structure has changed and continues to do so; an integrated delivery network spans hundreds of miles, and EPR information spans that same distance. With the implementation of HIPAA, vendors and users alike will go back to the drawing board to ensure that both access and security are addressed. It has been said that "privacy is the Achilles' heel of the information economy: the long-term winners will be players who make a firm, public, and unambiguous commitment to a strong set of privacy standards and stick to them. Not only is this the right thing to do, it is also the competitively advantaged strategy."[2]

The security section of the HIPAA regulations has not yet been finalized at the time of this writing; however, the final regulation is expected sometime in the near future. The proposed regulations are written to support the provider's ability to assess their own information security culture to determine where existing weaknesses lie and how to address those weaknesses. HIPAA is considered technology-neutral and does not require specific remedies to problems, but it does outline a variety of processes to be considered in achieving a more secure electronic environment.

The transactions and code-sets portion of the regulation has also been finalized and went into effect in October 2002, with a one-year deadline extension available on request, extending the effective date to October 2003. This part of the regulation sets a national standard for the electronic billing of claims and for the use of standardized classification systems. Again, the EPR system supports this process through the sharing of electronic information between the EPR and billing systems.

HIPAA is seen by some to be laying the groundwork for eventual federal regulations requiring the use of electronic record-keeping systems. The thinking is that HIPAA is setting the standard for protection now before future regulations are developed to demand that all health information be made available electronically to support the mobility and fast-paced needs of our society.

THE HIM PROFESSIONALS' ROLE
IN EPR SYSTEM DEVELOPMENT AND USE

HIM professionals play a key role in determining the design and structure of electronic patient record systems.

System Selection

Collectively, HIM professionals direct the vendor community to develop effective systems that promote the patient care process, are easily used, and provide appropriate levels of security to protect patient privacy. Within their own employment settings, HIM professionals must play a leading role in selecting the system that best meets their specific health information needs. In addition to having a strong knowledge of the technical aspects of EPR development, the HIM professional must also develop or provide input into the request for proposal (RFP) used to initially communicate user needs with the system vendors being considered in the project. The administration and medical staff of the facility will also need to be convinced that an EPR system can be a valuable tool in providing patient care, increasing operational efficiency, and creating an environment that supports the use of burgeoning health information technology. The value of the EPR and other advanced IT systems can be demonstrated through a cost-benefit analysis. No one is better prepared than a HIM professional within the organization to participate in this process.

Once the system has been selected, the HIM professional can assume one of many leadership roles during the implementation phase. EPR system administrators are generally HIM professionals with additional expertise in the use of technology. This does not necessarily mean that a specific educational background in information systems technology is required, but it can certainly be helpful. The desire to improve the process, along with an interest in technology, usually lays the groundwork for EPR system administrators. This individual should be prepared to educate end users on systems benefits and work with the leadership of the organization to develop policies and procedures that will encourage system acceptance. For, like any other change, there will be rough spots in the process. Users must be willing to accept that fact and understand that in the end they will benefit from the change. The system administrator must also embrace his or her role as a change agent in this process.

In widespread EPR systems, there is a marked need for training. This is often a full-time job and one that requires special skills in working with adult learners. HIM professionals again have demonstrated a clear ability to excel in these roles.

HIM professionals also commonly fill the role of report writer. Once the data are in the system, someone has to know how to get them out. Combined with the technical skill of computerized report processing, using SQL or some other reporting language the HIM professional can create reports and validate their accuracy.

Data Validation

Because of the intricacies involved with how information reaches the EPR system, there is a definite need to validate the data exchange process. Once an interface has been created, it cannot be assumed that it works. To prove the process is stable, validation programs must be developed and used. The HIM professional has traditionally been known to be particularly detail-oriented, and data validation requires just that skill. System testing should occur frequently to ensure that the information sent from one system is received in the appropriate form by the receiving system. Testing once is not enough; it must be repeated, even after the interface is being used in the production environment. This is necessary because any program change in the sending or receiving system (or anywhere in the send or translation process) may negatively affect the data exchange. For example, take the case of a respiratory therapy program that is upgraded to a newer version. Even though the identification fields in the respiratory system may appear to look exactly as they did in the previous version, a programming feature known as *truncation* may have been added. This means that the identification field may have been set for twenty characters in the respiratory system, but the new feature was added to cut off any blank spaces at the end of the identification number. This wouldn't seem to be a problem, as most identification numbers are from six to twelve characters in length. However, even though the spaces are blank in the respiratory system, the EPR system expects all twenty characters to be sent across. When the EPR system doesn't receive the anticipated information, system errors are generated.

HIM professionals are also well suited for creating and maintaining housewide data dictionaries. Again, because so many feeder systems supply information to the EPR, there is a need to understand what each field name means for each system. This is important in the data validation process as well. For example, let's assume that the nursing documentation system includes a field named "patient account number." That field is seven characters long and represents the unique visit detail for a specific patient. Let's further assume that the dietary system feeds data to the EPR also and that it includes a field named "patient identification." That field is six characters long and represents what the hospital information system and EPR system know to be a medical record number. This could cause great confusion, but with a standardized data dictionary for reference, all users are able to determine which information is needed, what the original source of those data is, and what the information really means.

Finally, with the advent of HIPAA and the increased demand for data security, HIM professionals often participate in system disaster recovery programs; they work in teams that address appropriate security levels. The assessment of biometric security methods like retinal or thumbprint scanning and physical security issues, the development of policies and procedures to ensure data security, and the coordination with IT department leadership to create a secure information environment are becoming increasingly prominent roles for HIM professionals as well.

CONCLUSION

The generation of health care providers who were unwilling to accept technological solutions for the documentation of patient health history and status is gradually leaving the workforce. User acceptance of technology is already becoming more widespread. And soon, not only will technology be accepted by users but it will be demanded. A clear example is the willingness of physicians to use personal digital assistants (PDAs). Known more broadly under the concept name of *palm technology,* these small and efficient pieces of equipment are appearing daily in the hands of health care providers. Many organizations have not been prepared to deal with the expanding security dilemmas created by the use of such equipment. Yet many physicians are using technology of this type to transfer data from the health care facility to their offices. Physicians are also finding significant benefit from PDAs in terms of their ability to facilitate the office billing practices. In fact, some believe that with the use of charge-capture software on a PDA, "five years from now in the smart [medical] practice, there won't be any accounts receivable follow-up as we know it today."[3]

In some cases, hospital policies have been developed to prohibit the use of such technology for fear that patient information is not being appropriately protected. Instead of banning the use of such equipment, more sophisticated security measures will have be developed to meet the market forces that are driving the change. The fact that physicians and other care providers are buying into that technology is a clear sign that automation is the way of the future.

Other current trends in automation include the growing acceptance of the use of electronic signatures at both state and national levels. Many states have laws regarding the allowable use of electronic signatures in general and in health care specifically. A federal law known as Electronic

Signatures in Global and National Commerce Act was enacted recently to support this concept as well.

The next generation of EPR systems will enjoy far greater use than their predecessors. The pioneers who moved information technology to the HIM forefront will see the fruits of their efforts more widely accepted and increasingly demanded. The HIM profession will continue to advocate the need for access, in balance with security, until finally the EPR will be the norm instead of the exception.

REFERENCES

1. www.its.bodrdoc.gov
2. P. Evans and T. Wurster, *Blown to Bits* (Boston: Harvard Business School Press, 2000): 167.
3. C. Toth, *The Journal of Medical Economics* (December 17, 2001): 50.

CHAPTER 4

Information-Capture Design and Principles

Linda S. Kiger

Health information management involves the total management of all data concerning a patient, including the control, organization, and collection of patient data and the creation of output from those data. Thus HIM professionals are responsible for ensuring the effective design and implementation of information-capture tools for data collection and use.

Well-designed health record documents, whether paper or electronic, are important communication tools as well as ready references for use in providing patient care and in reviewing the care provided. This chapter examines the principles of design for paper forms, computer-view design, and practice guidelines for information capture.

Practice Guidelines for Information Capture

Information-capture control objectives, according to the guidelines of AHIMA, include the following:

- Maximizing efficiency throughout the enterprise by the effective design and construction of paper forms and computer screens

- Establishing and controlling standards for information content and vocabulary

- Originating and maintaining proper specifications for information capture and usage

- Ensuring consistent and accurate capture, storage, and usage of information

- Streamlining the information-capture process by eliminating duplicate data entry, ensuring that information capture follows the flow of work, reducing key strokes, and ensuring that users have information when they need it

- Establishing institutionwide guidelines and criteria for the development and revision of information-capture tools.[1]

Health record forms are designed to facilitate data collection as well as to provide complete and accurate data. Whether the facility uses a paper-based patient record or a computer-based patient record, the same principles should be applied. (Note that using the CPR does not necessarily eliminate paper forms; paper may be used as an intermediary between the individual and the computer.) In this case, forms must also be carefully designed to ensure appropriate data collection and guidance for entering data into the computer.

As discussed in Chapter Two, neither the AHA nor the Joint Commission recommends any specific health record forms. Standards organizations such as the ASTM and AHIMA have not recommended forms or computer views with which to collect requisite data elements. As a result, each health care facility is free to adopt the information-capture tools that best meet its needs.

Ideally, HIM professionals should work with other health care professionals within the facility to develop forms that promote adherence to standards for documenting patient care, organize information for easy reference, reduce wasted space, and eliminate unnecessary duplication. In addition, forms should take into consideration the individual user's needs.

Thus they should be comprehensible to the staff members responsible for completing them and to the staff members who are guided by the recorded information in rendering patient care. For example, the summary sheet of the record may be designed to contain admission information, patient identification data, and consents and authorizations. This face sheet may also include information relative to diagnoses and procedures. The key factor is that the information be captured in the most efficient method for the health care facility.

In some communities, two or more health care facilities work together, through a representative committee, to adopt basic forms or documents that are acceptable to their medical and hospital staffs. This type of joint effort saves money by sharing printing costs. In addition, when physicians practice in more than one health care facility, the use of the same forms in several of the community's health care facilities simplifies the recording procedure and promotes adherence to high standards. A cooperative spirit among HIM professionals at different facilities also promotes the development of common forms and results in improved documentation. As an alternative, a health care corporation may design generic core forms or views for its entities, allowing local facilities to make necessary modifications.

A goal of the HIM professional in the area of information capture is to eliminate duplicative data, thus providing a succinct health record that reflects the high quality of care that is rendered. The principles of information capture discussed in this chapter apply to computer-generated forms and secondary forms, as well as to forms in the primary health record.

Role of the Forms Committee

Because the authority to enter information into the health record is granted by the medical staff, health record forms should be approved by a representative group of the medical staff—usually the medical record committee. This committee may act as a forms committee, or a separate forms committee may be appointed by the medical staff to maintain an effective form design and control program. The duties and authority of the forms committee should be clearly defined and supported by the health care facility's administration. The HIM department director may serve as chairperson of the forms committee to coordinate the tasks involved.

The committee reviews forms, recommends changes in content, makes design changes to conform to an established basic record format (for example, standard location and sequence of identifying information and standard margins), and eliminates unnecessary forms. When a separate forms committee handles forms review, a mechanism should be in place to facilitate feedback to the medical record committee for the coordination of tasks and communication of information relevant to the health record.

Traditionally, the forms committee develops, reviews, and controls all facilitywide information-capture tools. The committee should comprise information users and those responsible for entering documentation and should include representatives from health information management, the medical staff, nursing, purchasing, and information services.

A system for numbering forms allows easy identification and stock control. Kept on file are samples of all editions of approved forms. A brief statement of its purpose and principal uses accompanies each form. The form number and the approval date are printed on each revision. A list of these assigned form numbers, their titles, and the dates of approval for each is recommended. It also serves as a catalog. The health record forms numbering system should be coordinated with a facilitywide system for numbering forms.

Principles of Paper Form Design

When a new form is developed, it is advisable to prepare a small supply of forms for trial use because experience frequently indicates a need for revisions. Because cost is also a factor in continually revising and printing small quantities of forms, photocopying an initial supply might be the reproduction method of choice. Forms that become obsolete each year, such as a routing slip or charge ticket in a physician's office that lists diagnosis and procedure codes, should be ordered in quantities of no more than a year's supply. Old or discontinued forms should be removed from the stockroom or supply area and discarded.

A basic concept of form design is to keep forms simple and few in number to provide flexibility and to reduce record bulk. Before a new form is developed or an existing form is revised, the forms committee might review the steps in Figures 4.1 and 4.2 to compile the necessary facts and determine what, if any, improvements should be made.

The following principles are essential to good paper form design:

- A uniform size of paper is used. The standard $8\frac{1}{2}" \times 11"$ is the best size for a document.

- A uniform binding edge is maintained, along the top or the side. Optical character reader codes and bar codes are typically printed in the upper-left corner of the form.

- Uniform margins based on the binding edge are maintained. Chart holders on the nursing units should accommodate the uniform margins. Margins are at least 3/8" wide. If the document has punched holes, the margins are at least 3/4" wide.

- For top binding, information printed on two-sided forms is correctly placed on both sides for proper assembly in the chart. For side binding, the two sides are placed head-to-head.

- Vertical and horizontal lines are used to assist the user in completing and reviewing the form.

- The quality and weight of paper are selected according to the expected life of the record, the amount of use it will receive, and whether both sides are to be used. If both sides are printed, the paper is heavy enough to prevent any ink or copy from showing through one side to the other. A 20- to 24-pound stock is recommended for use in copiers, scanners, and fax machines.

Figure 4.1. Gathering the Facts to Design a New Information-Capture Tool

Need

- What procedures will be accomplished by completing this form? Will its use justify its existence?
- On what other forms is this information duplicated in part or completely?
- What inadequacies are there in completing this form or in performing the procedures?

Staff: Health Care Facility or Medical

- Who requires or wants this information in part or completely—medical staff, individual physicians, other professional staff, patient accounts, administration, outside agencies, payers?
- Who enters the information?
- Who will use this information? Is it used in original, abstracted, or statistical form?

Location

- Where is the form initiated, completed, and processed?
- Where is the form sent, and what is the distribution?
- Where is the form filed?

Time

- When is the information entered on the form?
- What causes delays in completing the form?
- Should the form be held in the unit pending completion?
- When is the form filed?

Method

- How are data entered on the form? Are they written or generated by a word processor, microprocessor, or mainframe computer?
- How is the information on this form distributed to other units that need the information, either whole or in part?
- How many units are maintaining files for part or all of the information on this form? How many duplicate forms are in departments of the facility?

Figure 4.2. Improving an Existing Information-Capture Tool

Need

- Is the proposed information needed?
- Does the cost of gathering or recording the information exceed the information's worth?
- Is there a more reliable source or an easier way to obtain the information?
- Can existing forms or any items on the form at hand be combined, eliminated, simplified, rearranged for better sequencing, or enlarged to accommodate additional items?

Staff: Health Care Facility or Medical

- Can the work of completing part or all of the form's data items be delegated to nonprofessional staff?
- Can the handling or processing of the form be done by other units or clerks to simplify the work? Can it be combined with other procedures for handling?
- Can the data items be re-sequenced or revised to simplify entering and recalling or abstracting the data?

Location

- Can the completion and processing of the form be done better in another unit or combined with similar work in another unit?
- Can the form be designed to eliminate the need to initiate another form, make copies of the completed form, or copy the information on another form?
- Can the form be designed better to facilitate filing, retrieval, storage, and retirement (disposal)?

Time

- Is there a more timely method for entering the information?
- Can peak loads be leveled off by better scheduling of procedures to complete and process information?
- Can a staff member be assigned to initiate the form by requesting information when it is available and then processing it during slack times?

Figure 4.2. Continued

Method

- Can the writing method be changed for ease and timeliness in completion?
- Can the routing method be improved?
- Has the form been developed to use the most efficient office equipment and to accommodate an integrated information system?
- Can authorized persons centralize the information in this form for access, thus eliminating the duplication of files?
- Is the design user-friendly?

- Color forms are carefully selected to prevent any problems in the future with photocopying, imaging, or faxing. Using white paper with black ink and color-coded borders is effective for quick identification of different forms in a hard-copy record; however, it is very expensive and therefore not cost-efficient.

- When feasible, using a rubber stamp on an existing form eliminates the need for a special form that is not used regularly.

- A typical font size is 12 points. For legibility, lowercase letters are at least 9 points in size and uppercase letters at least 10 points.

- Patient-identifying information such as name, Social Security number, health record number, physician name and number, and date of birth appear on every page.

- A signature line appears on every report to prevent questions about authentication.

Principles of Computer-View Design

Many of the previous principles also apply to computer-view design. However, some issues are unique to the computerization of data:

- *Control issues and confidentiality:* Access is limited to users who are authorized to view the information. Those who need to use the information should be able to easily retrieve it and enter new information, if necessary. Information stored in the computer must be captured, arranged, and available to the authorized user.

- *Efficient keyboarding:* Data are arranged to allow efficient data entry. The form should be arranged in a logical format. A data dictionary or catalog that contains definitions for all the entities and relationships will allow the user to enter information using a minimum number of strokes.

- *Correct formatting:* A computer screen only shows about one-third of a form at a time. It is therefore important that the data be efficiently organized so that the user can move immediately to the appropriate section without scrolling through many screens.

- *Cost considerations:* Computers can print volumes of paper each day, which may exceed the amount used in the traditional paper record. The forms committee or view management team needs to address this issue and develop an efficient system for the facility to print only what is necessary.

- *Standardized vocabularies:* A computer system demands standardized terminology, abbreviations, and definitions. Where standard definitions are not available, the computer view should supply the definition.

- *External standards:* Voluntary standard-setting groups such as the ASTM, Health Level Seven (HL7), and others are working to develop standards to facilitate the electronic interchange of information on admissions, discharges, and transfers within facilities. The ASTM standards are specifically designed to facilitate the creation of computer-based patient records. In particular, the ASTM standard E1384–99el, *Standard Guide for Content and Structure of the Electronic Health Record,* covers the following issues:[2]

- Identifying the content and logical structure of a computer-based patient record

- Defining the relation of data coming from diverse source systems and the data stored in the CPR

- Providing a common vocabulary, perspective, and references for those developing, purchasing, and implementing CPR systems

- Describing examples of a variety of views by which the logical data structure might be accessed or displayed to accomplish various functions

- Relating the logical structure of the CPR to the essential documentation currently used in the health care delivery system in the United States to promote consistency and efficient data transfer

Principles of Information Capture

The following principles are basic to good tools for information capture, whether the document is paper or computerized:

- The need and purpose for every item on the form is demonstrated. (Items that "might be nice to have" or "may be needed some day" require collection time that is disproportionate to the value of the information.)

- Items are listed in logical sequence. (For example, it is logical to place age immediately following date of birth and telephone number following address.)

- The spaces allowed for computerized entries accommodate the font selected for printing.

- Spacing is planned according to the method of documentation, whether computerized or handwritten.

- All forms display the patient's identification in a standard location.

- When uniform placement is not feasible, common items on related forms follow a uniform sequence.

- Terminology in item headings is consistent on all forms.

- Forms that require a transfer of information from other parts of the record are avoided.

- The name of the facility is preprinted on all forms to identify any authorized photocopies used outside the health care facility. (To save space, the name can be placed sideways in the left margin of the form.)

- In certain areas of the document, the use of bold print for emphasis can be effective.

- For easy identification, a document number and revision date appear on each form.

- Forms provide instructions on how they are to be completed. (Instructions are placed on the top, in small print, whenever possible. Routing instructions are placed at the bottom. If symbols or abbreviations are used, a legend is included, which is typically found in the upper-left corner.)

- Answer boxes save time in completing the form and reduce errors, and they provide uniformity for statistical items. (However, the item must be explicit enough to make check-off or fill-in responses meaningful.)

- Multipart forms are considered whenever it is determined that a number of functions can be served by a single entry. The additional cost of the form is weighed against other items, such as the cost of handling extra forms or making duplicate entries.

Duplicating Systems

The nature of the systems available for making copies of health record forms pertains to the process of information capture and design. A few available options include making carbon copies, using continuous forms, using standing-order forms, and making photocopies.

Carbonizing

Carbon copies of forms can be made by inserting loose carbon sheets between blank forms or by using form pads with carbons already inserted. Snap-out forms with a one-use carbon are also available. No-carbon-required (NCR) forms have replaced loose carbon sheets almost entirely, however. The chemically treated paper used for NCR forms permits reproduction of the documentation on one or more copies in a set of forms without the use of carbon paper. A problem with NCR sheets, however, is that they cannot be placed between other forms still in use in the health record.

Using Continuous Forms

Word processing units for transcribing histories and physical examination reports, discharge summaries, and other dictation can use continuous forms. The transcriptionist can type on continuous forms that are later separated for filing into the patient's record. These forms are often preprinted with the health care facility's name or some other kind of identifying information. Because preprinted forms are expensive, another option is to type the information on a word processing template containing the standard wording and information.

Using Standing-Order Forms

A clinical service or a physician may request that the health care facility prepare quantities of physician order sheets with printed standing orders and blank space left for dosages of listed medications. Pharmacies generate such forms by computer. The physician then either enters the dosages on the forms or calls them in and signs the standing order. Such requests are made in the interest of starting care immediately after the patient's admission. The medical record committee or another appropriate medical staff committee approves requests for printed standing-order forms before the standing orders are printed.

Photocopying Forms

Photocopying is the easiest method available to produce multiple copies of a document, but it may also be the most expensive. Photocopy machines typically exist throughout the health facility and vary a great deal in features and use. The HIM department uses photocopiers extensively and requires machines with such features as two-sided copying, collating, and reducing or enlarging. It may choose to sign a service contract with an outside vendor to handle the majority of its copying workload, at a pre-established rate. Employees of the service then work in the health care facility.

Secondary disclosure of health record information is of paramount concern to the HIM professional. When copies of part or all of a patient's health record are made and forwarded to individuals or organizations outside the health care facility, a label (either stamped or permanently affixed) should be secured on one or more sheets stating that any disclosure of health record information by the recipient(s) is prohibited except when implicit in the purposes of this disclosure. No more patient information should be copied than is necessary to carry out the purpose of the disclosure.

Conclusion

All aspects of information capture continue to challenge the HIM professional. Health records have traditionally been paper documents, and it is anticipated that some paper will still exist once the vast majority of records have been computerized. However, computerization links patient information, whether it is kept in traditional health record paper forms or in a network server throughout the enterprise. In either format, the HIM professional lends form expertise, as well as knowledge of information flow within a health care facility, to help in the design and maintenance of the optimal system. Well-designed forms and computer information systems are a key to efficient and effective data communication, with the ultimate benefit of high-quality patient care.

REFERENCES

1. AHIMA, Practice Brief, "Practice Guidelines for Managing Health Information," *Journal of AHIMA* 68, no. 3 (March 1997).
2. American Society for Testing and Materials Sub-Committee E31.19, *Guide E1384–99e1 Standard Guide for Content and Structure of the Electronic Health Record (EHR)* (West Conshohocken, Penn.: ASTM, 2001).

WEB SITES

www.ahima.org

www.astm.org

CHAPTER 5

Health Record Analysis

Nancy Coffman-Kadish

A s discussed in earlier chapters, the patient health record is a compilation of general and specialized health record forms and documents that contain specific patient care information. To help ensure that the health record and its component forms and documents are complete, the HIM department may conduct an analysis, or review, of the record. This chapter describes the traditional, detailed approach to health record review (performed after patient discharge) and the newer, more focused and concurrent approach (performed during the patient's stay in the institution).

It is important to note that in reviewing the health record for documentation adequacy, the HIM professional does not render judgments or assessments regarding the quality of care. That task is performed by peer groups of health care providers. However, the HIM professional's review of documentation plays an important role in the assessment of clinical quality. Such evaluations of record thoroughness, timeliness, and accuracy indicate the degree to which it will be useful for gauging the quality of care provided. A complete record also supports patient care and expedites the billing process.

MAJOR STEPS IN HEALTH RECORD ANALYSIS

Health record analysis, sometimes known as *discharge analysis* or *postdischarge analysis,* refers to the tasks involved in processing the health records of discharged patients. Health record analysis helps to ensure that records are complete, accurate, timely, and legible, and that patterns of documentation among physicians and other health care providers are noted and assessed. Major tasks typically performed during the analysis include review of admission, discharge, and transfer reports; assembly of forms and documents within the health record folder; and quantitative and qualitative analysis of record contents.

Tasks Associated with the Admission, Discharge, and Transfer Report

To track patients, health care facility information systems generate a daily admission, discharge, and transfer (ADT) report, which is a list of patients who have been admitted, discharged (including those who have died), or transferred from one bed or unit to another. The ADT report lists patients by name, bed number or location, and health record number. This list is distributed internally to the HIM department and to various other departments.

An accurate ADT report is an essential tool for many HIM departments performing quality assessments. The HIM department uses its copy of the ADT as a checklist to ensure that all records of discharges and deaths have been received or otherwise accounted for. Records of previous admissions that have been forwarded to the nursing station for review during care must also be returned to the HIM department for proper filing. Furthermore, the computerized or manual master patient index (MPI) must be updated to reflect recent discharges, deaths, and transfers.

Record Assembly

Upon a patient's discharge, HIM department staff may assemble the patient's health record in an established order. Patient records at the nurses' station are typically maintained in reverse-chronological order to facilitate continuous updating and reference requirements. After the patient is discharged, the HIM department staff member may reassemble the record in an established sequence that is more conducive to future, ongoing use. The established order is one accepted by the medical staff (or its medical record committee), in cooperation with the health care facility administration. It is often referred to as the *chart order* or *health record format* for permanent filing. The patient record typically also includes any ambulatory care or outpatient services forms within this single, or unit, record.

The word *permanent* refers to the length of time that health records are to be maintained in their original or nonminiaturized form. The health record is kept in the permanent active file until it is scanned, microfilmed, placed in an inactive file, or properly destroyed after the required retention period.

The permanent health record is arranged in its component parts (medical, ancillary services, and nursing), with either reverse chronological or chronological filing within each component, usually according to the source-oriented format. (Recall from Chapter Two that in the source-oriented format, each department documents care within its own section of the record.) If the integrated format is used, all forms are organized in date order, and those from various sources are intermingled. No matter what format is selected, the format should promote an ease of referencing needed information.

To save time and money, some health care facilities choose to perform a modified assembly or not to reassemble the record at all. In a modified system, major sections are assembled, but a strict date order is not required. If the health care facility chooses not to reassemble the record after patient discharge, it is said to be using a *universal chart order*. This means that the medical staff, nursing, and the HIM and other involved departments have agreed on an order that is used while the patient is in-house; the order will remain the same after discharge, including for permanent filing. When a universal chart order is used, two options are available for the HIM department in handling the record after discharge. The first is to file the record exactly as it is received from the unit. The unit clerk is usually responsible for ensuring that the record is in the agreed-upon order and for removing any unnecessary forms or copies. The other option is for the HIM department staff to verify the order and remove any copies or unnecessary forms. The HIM department staff also reviews each form and report in the record to ensure that it belongs to the indicated patient. The assembly method that is chosen depends on anticipated needs for future retrieval of the information.

Overview of Quantitative Analysis

Quantitative analysis is conducted to determine the accuracy and completeness of the health record. HIM professionals who have oversight responsibility for assembling the records of discharged patients perform a quantitative analysis function to determine the presence or absence of essential reports and items such as the following:

- Discharge summary or clinical résumé
- History and physical examination report (H&P)
- Authentication (signatures) for designated entries in the health record (for example, progress notes, physician's orders, and operative reports)
- Principal and additional diagnoses and principal and additional procedures documented by the attending physician
- Operative report, preanesthesia and postanesthesia reports, and pathology report for patients requiring surgery
- Reports of all diagnostic tests or studies ordered (for example, laboratory, radiology, EEG, and EKG)
- Authenticated consultation reports (if a consultation was requested)
- Signed authorizations and consents
- Correct patient identification on every paper form or computer screen

- Complete and authenticated reports that are required for patients in units such as obstetrics, neonatal, and rehabilitation

A more detailed description of the documents and data collected during the quantitative analysis appears later in this chapter.

Deficiency Systems. To note the absence of materials or items, the HIM professional may use a manual or a computerized deficiency system. With the manual system, the HIM professional compares the contents of the health record with a checklist. Should reports or signatures be missing, the HIM professional tags the health record folder with a slip that specifies the deficiencies and the physicians or staff members who are responsible for correcting them. Missing signatures are typically indicated in the record with a colored clip or tag, with the color indicated next to the responsible physician's name on the deficiency slip. When the record is completed, the slip is removed and discarded.

With a computerized deficiency system, the deficiencies are entered into a computer using a specialized program. The program tracks the deficiencies for each record, which is updated as the deficiencies are completed. The program also tracks the number and types of deficiencies by physician. Most programs also generate the reminder letters sent out at predetermined intervals, notifying the physicians of any incomplete or delinquent medical records. Management reports are available that indicate the deficiencies by type (for example, missing discharge summaries, missing physician order signatures) and number. Reports can list responsible physicians by name, with the type and number of deficiencies for each.

Implementation of an electronic health record drastically changes these functions. Record assembly is no longer performed. Quantitative analysis is still necessary, but the authentication of reports is changed. Software for maintaining electronic records contains documentation prompts, built-in edits, and other mechanisms designed to ensure that the record is complete at the point of data entry.

Deficiency Follow-Up Activities. Often the HIM professional must follow up on deficiencies identified during the analysis process. For example, he or she may investigate late or missing diagnostic reports, or examine specific issues (for example, problems on the nursing unit in entering patients' reports into the health records) during department or institution-wide quality-assessment studies. In addition, the HIM department director should prepare a weekly (or biweekly) report that indicates the number of incomplete and delinquent medical records, the type and number of deficiencies, and the physicians responsible for correcting them. It is also good practice to closely monitor the length of time that each record has remained incomplete. This report is then distributed to the respective physicians, the medical record committee, the chief of the medical staff, and the health care facility administrator or vice president to whom the HIM director reports.

Overview of Qualitative Analysis

Qualitative analysis is the process involved in checking the content of the health record to identify inconsistent or inaccurate documentation. Thus the record is reviewed for accuracy and adherence to documentation procedures and standards rather than for the presence or absence of forms and signatures. As a result of the review, the record is found to be complete and accurate or incomplete and inaccurate.

Qualitative Analysis and the Quality Assessment Study. Often the qualitative review is the by-product of quality activities that are performed to assess patient care. For example, HIM professionals who assist the medical staff in abstracting the health record for compliance with quality-of-care criteria sometimes find that the recorded information is inadequate for the purpose. This discovery prompts an investigation into the reasons for the inadequacy. The findings of the investigation can be useful to the medical record committee and the quality assessment committee in promoting better documentation in the health record.

Qualitative Review Checklist. Another approach to qualitative analysis is to develop a checklist of significant points to be reviewed for documentation. Such a list might be developed by the HIM professional in cooperation with the medical record committee or a representative group of the medical staff and other professional staff. The following list provides examples of questions asked in the qualitative review of health records:

- Does the admitting process consistently and accurately gather demographic data for inclusion in the patient health record?

- Does the history of present illness reflect the patient's own words?

- Does the patient's history include references to any past problems or to problems in the family history? Does it include a review of body systems as required in the criteria established for qualitative review?

- Do physicians' orders reflect the clinical problem for which each service or item is ordered? Is there evidence that every order was carried out?

- Do the physician's progress notes describe the patient's problems, his or her clinical state of comfort or distress, and the reasons behind the therapeutic decisions?

- What is the turnaround time, or TAT as it is commonly referred to, of the dictated reports? TAT is the time lapse between dictation and transcription of the H&P, operative reports, and other dictated reports. Do the reports reflect the dates of both dictation and transcription?

- Do the nurses' notes meet the criteria established for quality review of documentation? Are there time gaps in the record, or does the record reflect the general location of the patient at all times during the hospitalization?

- Are the health care facility guidelines for error correction followed?

- Are the rules for using symbols and abbreviations followed?

- Are there inconsistencies in the diagnoses noted throughout the record on the admitting forms, H&P report, operative report, pathology report, and discharge summary or clinical résumé?

- Does the patient's pharmacy drug profile match with the medication administered to the patient?

- Does the record reflect the discharge instructions given to the patient or the patient's family member, as well as the patient's or family member's understanding of these instructions?

By answering these and other questions, the HIM professional can pinpoint problems, such as the need for better information-capture tools, faster TAT in transcription, and corrective action in documentation.

Documents and Data Reviewed During Analysis

As described in the previous overviews of quantitative and qualitative analysis, the HIM professional checks a variety of documents for their level of completeness and accuracy during these two types of review. The subsections that follow highlight specific documents and data collected or reviewed during both processes.

Admission Records. The front sheet, also known as the top or face sheet, of the patient record contains a variety of information. Information entered by the admitting department and contained in the patient identification section of the front sheet varies in amount and specificity among health care facilities. The basic patient data that are required include name, address, health record number, age, date of birth, sex, race, marital status, religious preference, name of nearest relative, and nearest relative's address and telephone number. Also included on the front sheet are the admission date, room location or nursing unit assignment, source of payment, attending physician's name, type of admission, and admitting diagnosis or diagnoses. The HIM department may eventually add the discharge date, and any transfer of physician or clinical service may be noted as it occurs during hospitalization. For emergency admissions, the admitting staff does not always have access to all patient identification information. Missing information is added as it is received.

In addition, all pages of the health record must identify the patient by name, health record number, and nursing unit or room number. Typically, this information is computer-generated and printed on each form as it is produced.

The Discharge Summary and the Transfer Summary. The discharge summary, also called the clinical résumé, is a concise recapitulation of the patient's course in the health care facility. According to the Joint Commission, the discharge summary should contain the following items:

- Reason for hospitalization
- Significant findings
- Procedures performed and treatment rendered
- Patient's condition at discharge
- Instructions to the patient and family, if any[1]

All relevant diagnoses established during the course of care, as well as all operative and other invasive procedures that are performed, must be documented. This documentation must be entered in acceptable disease and operative terminology that includes etiology. A final progress note may be substituted for the clinical résumé for normal newborns with uncomplicated deliveries or patients with minor medical problems who require less than a forty-eight-hour period of hospitalization. The medical staff defines what medical conditions or problems are considered minor. The progress note may be handwritten or dictated. A discharge summary or final progress note must be completed and signed within thirty days of patient discharge.

It is imperative that the physician document the principal diagnosis, secondary diagnoses, principal procedure, and additional procedures in each record before the record is coded. If the diagnosis or procedure is not listed but is substantiated in the record, it must also be documented. The HIM professional must refer to the physician for clarification of any record in which a listed diagnosis or procedure is not substantiated or documented.

Although no accreditation standards or federal regulations have a specific time requirement for completion of the discharge summary, it should be noted that the entire record must be completed within thirty days of discharge. Therefore, hospital policy should specify a timeframe for completion of the discharge summary that will facilitate completion of the record within the thirty-day requirement.

In some facilities, physicians may have the option of contracting with outside services offered by health care professionals, such as credentialed HIM professionals, who dictate the requisite information for the discharge summary. The physician then attests to the accuracy of the information by signing the summary. This system, which reduces the amount of time required to enter the discharge summary onto the record, is made possible when the record contains sufficient information for the HIM professional to perform the dictation.

Discharge instructions provided to the patient or family may relate to physical activity, medication, diet, and follow-up care. A copy of diet instructions that are provided to the patient is entered into the health record or maintained on file in the health record department for reference as necessary. A copy of the discharge plan that is prepared by the social service department is also included in the health record.

When a patient is transferred within the same organization from one level of care to another, such as from acute care to a long-term care unit, a transfer summary may be substituted for the discharge summary. The transfer summary should briefly describe the patient's condition at the time of the transfer and the reason for the transfer. When the caregivers remain the same, a progress note may suffice.

History and Physical Examination. The patient history consists of the patient's chief complaint, a history of the present illness, relevant past medical, social, and family history, and a review of body systems. The physical examination should reflect a comprehensive, current physical assessment of the patient. The Joint Commission requires that the H&P examination be performed and documented by the examining physician within twenty-four hours of admission. If a complete history and physical examination was performed within thirty days before admission, a durable, legible copy of this report may be used in the patient's health record, provided that any changes that may have occurred are recorded in the health record at the time of admission. A durable, legible copy of the office prenatal or antepartum record is acceptable for obstetrical records.

An interval H&P note is included in the record when a patient is readmitted within thirty days of discharge for the same or a related condition. The interval notation should describe any changes in health status since the previous complete history and physical was documented. The original H&P must be available for the physician. If the readmission is for a different condition, a new H&P should be recorded.

The medical staff is responsible for determining those non-inpatient services such as ambulatory surgery for which a patient must have an H&P documented. Timely documentation of histories and physicals is important, whether the documentation is for an inpatient or an outpatient service.

Consultation Reports. A consultation is usually initiated by a written order or request from the attending physician to another physician or specialty department. The request states the purpose and the nature of the consultation that is desired. The consultation report should include evidence of a review of the patient's record, evidence of examination of the patient, pertinent findings of the examination, the consultant's opinion, diagnosis, or impression, and recommendations for treatment. A consultation may take the form of a separate consultation report or progress note; however, special forms are often used for certain types of examinations and tests, such as psychological tests. Copies of the consultation report are typically provided to the requesting physician and the consultant; the original is placed in the patient's health record.

Operative Reports. The preoperative diagnosis is entered in the record before surgery by the surgeon. Operative reports must be dictated or written immediately after surgery; they must contain the name of the primary surgeon and assistants, findings, technical procedures used, specimens removed, and the postoperative diagnosis. The completed operative report is signed by the surgeon and filed in the health record as soon as possible after surgery. If a resident serves as the assistant surgeon and dictates the operative report, the primary surgeon is still responsible for authenticating it. When a transcription or filing delay occurs in the HIM department, a comprehensive operative progress note is entered in the health record immediately after surgery to provide pertinent information for use by any individual who is required to attend to the patient.

Anesthesia Records. A preanesthesia evaluation must be completed within forty-eight hours prior to surgery by an individual qualified to administer anesthesia. This evaluation includes at least a review of objective diagnostic data, an interview with the patient to discuss his or her medical, anesthetic, and drug history, and a review of the patient's physical and emotional status.

The anesthesia record describes the monitoring of the patient, the dosage of all drugs and agents used, the type and amount of all fluids administered, including blood and blood products, the technique or techniques used, unusual events that occur during the anesthesia period, and the status of the patient at the conclusion of anesthesia. The anesthesia record must be signed by the anesthesiologist or anesthetist. Any unusual events or postoperative complications that arise, as well as the management of those events, must be recorded. The postoperative status of the patient is evaluated and documented on admission to and discharge from the postanesthesia care unit (PACU).

Progress Notes. Progress notes—signed, dated entries reflecting the course of the patient's illness or injury during hospitalization—are the responsibility of the physician(s) and other authorized staff members. The frequency with which progress notes are written depends on the patient's condition and the requirements of medical staff's rules or guidelines. The health care facility may establish guidelines for the handling of records that do not contain progress notes regarding patients who are hospitalized for more than a specified number of hours. In such cases, the records should be reviewed by the medical record or quality improvement committee. The clinical pertinence review, which is a medical staff responsibility delegated to the HIM department, may also identify such documentation problems.

As noted in earlier chapters, the Joint Commission has changed some of its requirements for authentication of some entries in the medical record. The Joint Commission does not specifically require signatures on progress notes, but the Medicare Conditions of Participation (COP) currently requires "prompt" authentication of health record entries, and individual state regulations may do so as well.

In the event of complicated hospital stays, progress notes must identify the complications and indicate the procedures and tests that are initiated, the types of problems being evaluated or ruled out, and the patient's response to the treatment modalities. The physician's progress notes should reflect a review of the documentation that is prepared by nurses and allied health practitioners.

Physician Orders. Physician orders direct a patient's diagnostic and therapeutic course in the health care facility. Diagnostic and therapeutic orders are dated and authenticated by the responsible practitioner. Verbal or telephone orders are acceptable only if allowed in the medical staff rules and regulations and if accepted and transcribed by qualified personnel, as identified by title or category in the medical staff rules and regulations. The medication orders of unlicensed interns and residents may require countersignatures by a medical staff member. The medical staff should have a written list of orders that require authentication by the responsible physician within a designated timeframe. The Joint Commission no longer requires physician signatures on verbal orders, except those for medication ordered in behavioral health care. Note, however, that authentication is required by the Medicare Conditions of Participation (COP) and may be required by other accreditation agencies or by state laws and regulations. The HIM professional should work with the health care institution to develop organizationwide policies to ensure compliance with legal, regulatory, and accreditation requirements.

Pathology and Clinical Laboratory Reports. The signed and dated original reports of pathology examinations and laboratory tests must also be placed in the health record. When tests are performed by outside laboratory services contracted by the health care facility, the name of the laboratory should be identified on the report placed in the patient's health record. The pathologist, in cooperation with the medical staff, decides which cases are exceptions to the rule that all specimens removed at surgery must be submitted to the pathology laboratory; exceptional specimens require only gross description and diagnosis. The HIM department should be aware of these exceptions. Most surgical pathology reports incorporate both gross and microscopic descriptions, with an accompanying diagnosis.

When an autopsy is performed, provisional anatomic diagnoses are typically recorded in the health record within three days, and a complete protocol should be made a part of the record within sixty days, unless exceptions for special studies are established by the medical staff. Data collected from autopsies should be shared with those responsible for improving health care facility performance. The data collection process itself must be guided by clear assessment criteria.

Radiological and Other Diagnostic Reports. Signed and dated original radiological reports, as well as other diagnostic reports, are also filed in the health record. The practitioner who interprets the film, tracing, scan, ultrasound, or other image authenticates the report. Only those individuals with delineated clinical privileges for interpreting diagnostic studies or performing therapeutic, invasive procedures are authorized to authenticate reports of studies and procedures. Any reports on preadmission diagnostic procedures should accompany the admission record to the nursing unit.

Medication Administration Records. The medication administration record (MAR) provides documentation of the medicines administered orally or topically or by infusion, inhalation, or injection. The date, time, name of drug, dose, route, and signature or initials of the individual who administered the drug must be documented. Adverse drug reactions must also be documented in accordance with facility policies and procedures.

Nursing Records. Clinical nursing records consist of information on patient assessments, nursing care plans, nursing diagnoses or patient needs, nursing interventions, and patient outcomes. The patient's health record includes documentation of the nursing care that is provided, as well as the patient's response to it and to all other care. Nursing documentation includes many forms and formats, such as narrative notes, flowcharts, questionnaires, checklists, and graphics. Nursing forms may be paper-based, computerized, or a combination of the two.

Nursing documentation in the health record should be pertinent and concise, and it should reflect the patient's status. In so doing, it documents the patient's needs, problems, capabilities, and limitations. The patient assessment—an important part of nursing documentation—is performed either at the time of admission or within a period preceding or following admission that is specified in the health care facility policy. The Joint Commission requires that the nursing assessment be completed within twenty-four hours of admission. The assessment includes consideration of biophysical, psychosocial, environmental, self-care, educational, and discharge planning factors.

When the patient is transferred to another nursing unit or is discharged from the health care facility, a nurse documents the patient's present status in the health record. The record also reflects any discharge instructions provided to the patient or the patient's representative.

Usually, the health care facility's established policy on nursing reports dictates the frequency and method of recording information. Forms to facilitate nursing documentation have check columns for routine services rendered. Nursing notes may be documented on nursing forms. Alternatively, a system of integrated progress notes may be used. In this system, all health care practitioners document patient care on a universal form (see Chapter Two).

Nursing care plans may be maintained separately from the patient health record at the nursing unit, and this information may or may not become a part of the health record. If the necessary information is recorded elsewhere in the record, the care plans may be retained temporarily (as determined by health care facility policy) and then destroyed. If the information documented in the care plan is not a recapitulation of information reflected in the record, the care plan becomes a part of the patient's permanent health record.

Therapy Reports. Therapy services are provided to the patient on physician order. Services provided must be accordance with the written plan of treatment. The original reports of the evaluation, recommendations, progress, and outcome of therapy department personnel, such as physical, respiratory, occupational, or speech, are to be included in the patient's health record.

Case Management or Social Service Reports. Case management or social service reports often contain sensitive details of the patient's personal life. Because some of this information might be of a hearsay nature that could be prejudicial to the patient or misinterpreted at a later date, the health care facility may prefer to have the social service department prepare an interpretative summary for the patient's record. The summary contains only that information of value to the physician and other professionals contributing to the patient's care. The sensitive information is then retained in the social service department's files.

Dietary Services. Like other members of the health care team, the dietitian cooperates by implementing the written orders of the attending physician. Each patient's nutritional care is planned, and an interdisciplinary nutrition therapy plan is developed and periodically updated for patients who are at nutritional risk.

The dietitian is required to promptly record in the patient's health record any pertinent, meaningful observations and information on the patient's food habits, food acceptance, and nutritional care plan. Whether the traditional source-oriented record format or the problem-oriented format is used, the health record entries should be timely, well organized, definitive, and amenable to the evaluation of the nutritional needs of the patient. The Joint Commission standards specify documentation requirements for nutrition services.

Federal and State Requirements for Record Content. In addition to the Joint Commission standards on record content that were described earlier, health care facilities must also adhere to federal and state requirements for health record content. As noted in some of the proceeding sections, health care facilities licensed to accept federal reimbursement must also meet the Medicare Conditions of Participation (COP) that are administered by the Centers for Medicare and Medicaid Services (CMS). The fiscal intermediary in each state can provide copies of the federal legislation that affects the health information system.

Each state board or department of health may have specific regulations that pertain to health record documentation. State regulations are usually available from the state's department of public health or other entity responsible for the licensure of health care facilities.

CONTEMPORARY TRENDS IN HEALTH RECORD ANALYSIS

The traditional, detailed review of the health record after discharge affords certain advantages. The chief advantage is that the HIM professional can perform a careful review of the record as a whole. A disadvantage of the discharge analysis is that it can delay the completion or correction of documentation, which can then adversely affect patient care. One might question, for example, whether it is ethical to sign orders after a patient is discharged and how such a practice benefits the patient's care. One might also wonder what effect such unsigned orders may have on the health care facility's potential liability for a negative patient outcome. Clearly, retrospective documentation does not add value to patient care. In recognition of this fact, AHIMA has developed a position statement that supports the need for clinical information to be made available at the point of care for clinical decision making. The recommendation is that health care practitioners record their findings at the point of care or within twenty-four hours of an encounter.[2]

Another disadvantage of the traditional discharge analysis is that it can hinder the billing process because the coding and sequencing of diagnoses and procedures cannot be performed until the requisite documentation is entered in the record. When the HIM department has to wait for documentation to be completed in order to code data and submit the record to the business office, the financial impact on the health care facility is significant. To facilitate the billing process, many health care facilities require immediate completion of some parts of the record after discharge but are willing to modify completion requirements in other areas. In addition, many HIM departments have changed the traditional sequence of postdischarge processing of the record from assembly, then analysis, and then coding to coding first, then assembly and analysis. This sequence facilitates timely coding, and thus the bill can be submitted more promptly.

A final drawback of traditional discharge analysis is the amount of time that is required to perform tasks such as reviewing records for omissions, notifying physicians of needed information, counting delinquent records, and pursuing late documentation. From the HIM professional's point of view, this time might be better spent managing, analyzing, and presenting health data, planning and implementing the computerization of records, and assessing and meeting customer needs.

Health Information Management

For all these reasons, the focus of contemporary health record practice has begun to shift from detailed discharge analysis to either a more simplified approach or concurrent analysis. In an attempt to operate more efficiently, some health care facilities have also sought to streamline the analysis process or adopt a more focused type of health record review.

Concurrent Analysis

In the concurrent approach to the health record review, the HIM professional performs quantitative and qualitative analysis on the nursing units while the patient is still hospitalized. (Workspace for this type of analysis must be provided at or near the nursing station.) Reviews of the record are performed daily to identify deficiencies and to notify the staff members who are responsible for correcting them. The goal of concurrent analysis is to make the record as complete as possible while the patient is in the facility receiving care, so as to improve documentation and, ultimately, patient care.

When the concurrent approach is used, other record processing functions may be performed at the remote location as well. The record may be assembled in permanent filing order, completed, abstracted, coded, and assigned a DRG within a few hours of the patient's discharge. Final record processing and permanent filing still take place in the HIM department.

The Electronic Signature and Other Streamlining Techniques

Traditionally, HIM professionals have gone to great lengths during the analysis process to secure the physician's signature on various reports in the health record. Signatures have been sought on dictated reports such as the H&P, operative report, and the clinical résumé. The electronic signature, which has been approved by the Joint Commission and is acceptable under the Medicare Conditions of Participation, has eliminated much of the tagging and flagging associated with the health record in the past.

Electronic signatures incorporate the dictation system's physician identifier code that is the key to his or her dictation of patient health record documents. In such a system, each individual who is authorized to use the dictation system has an assigned security code. To gain access to the system, the physician must enter his or her unique identification code. To maintain security and meet Joint Commission standards, every physician participating in the electronic signature program must be required to sign a participation form verifying that he or she is the only individual with access to that unique physician signature code and is the only one who will use it.

The responsible health care practitioner signs the record entry by entering a unique code or password that verifies his or her identity. A statement may appear on the document, such as "electronically signed by Alex Smith, MD," with the date and time noted. The Joint Commission requires that the computer system allow the author to review the document online before signing electronically. Therefore, before the electronic signature is applied, the physician should have an opportunity to review a hard copy or an on-line version of the document and to revise the document, correct any errors, or enter any missing data.

Simplified Deficiency Processing

In addition to the electronic signature, other streamlining techniques have eliminated the flagging of orders or progress notes with missing signatures after discharge. Health care facilities that follow one or more of these practices may nevertheless retain requirements in key areas, such as requiring authentication on the history and physical examinations, operative reports, consultations, and discharge summaries, as required by the Joint Commission.

With simplified deficiency processing, retrospective chart analysis still occurs but in a reduced form. Only those items identified as critical are analyzed for completeness.[3] This method is effective only if all concerned parties are in agreement and if the medical staff is educated about the limits of retrospective review and their responsibilities regarding timely documentation and authentication. Continued monitoring of the critical deficiencies is important, with feedback provided to the medical staff departments and individual members.

Records may be marked "as is" and placed in the permanent file, even when there are deficiencies in the H&P, operative reports, or other pertinent dictated reports. For example, a timeframe (such as forty-five days) could be established to provide the physician ample opportunity to complete the chart. If the record is not completed in the specified timeframe, it is then filed "as is."

The Focused Review

Another example of operational efficiency is the focused review. The traditional discharge analysis requires a review of each item or form in the record for its completeness after patient discharge. In the focused review, a sample of records is evaluated for the presence or absence of crucial elements, as determined by the department or service. These elements differ by their relative importance to the department or service. The key to the effectiveness of the focused review is feedback to committees and medical staff departments. Results of the focused reviews are tabulated, analyzed, and presented. The departments and committees are responsible for developing action plans to resolve the problems at the point of documentation rather than correct them after patient discharge. Concurrent analysis can be accomplished while the patient record is on the floor if specific problems are identified in the focused review.

AHIMA published a practice brief titled "Best Practices in Medical Record Documentation and Completion"[4] to assist HIM professionals in making improvements in their facilities. This practice brief provides a table of best practices in the areas of documentation and chart completion. It would be available as long as it is deemed current at the AHIMA Web site at www.ahima.org.

In addition, AHIMA has challenged its members to work together to prevent incomplete health records instead of concentrating on delinquencies.[5] AHIMA is continuing to work with the Joint Commission in the management of information standards. The challenge for the HIM professional is to devise methodologies that improve the documentation system as a whole—not just the individual record.

The HIM professional is responsible for helping the health care facility move away from the detailed postdischarge analysis to a system that captures key health information concurrent with the patient stay. The health care provider is responsible for accurately and completely documenting the events of the patient's stay, but the HIM professional bears the responsibility for assisting in the development and maintenance of a health information system that facilitates this documentation.

CONCLUSION

Health record analysis has been a key function of HIM departments since the beginning of the health management profession. Today, however, the focus of the HIM professional has shifted from treating delinquencies to preventing incomplete health records. A record that is complete and produced on a timely basis is not the responsibility of the HIM professional alone but of all who record information in it. Complete information is integral to improving the quality of care rendered at the institution, facilitating the billing process, and allowing the HIM professional to perform the crucial functions of managing, analyzing, and presenting health care data.

REFERENCES

1. Joint Commission on Accreditation of Healthcare Organizations, *2001 Comprehensive Accreditation Manual for Hospitals* (Oakbrook Terrace, Ill.: Joint Commission, 2001).
2. AHIMA, Practice Brief, "Documentation Requirements for the Acute Care Inpatient Record," *Journal of AHIMA* (March 2001).
3. D. Grzybowski, "Simplified Deficiency Processing Brings Hospital-wide Benefits." *Journal of AHIMA* 71, no. 3 (March 2000): 58–61.
4. AHIMA, Practice Brief, "Best Practices in Medical Record Documentation and Completion," *Journal of AHIMA* (November/December 1999).
5. AHIMA, Practice Brief, "Authentication of Medical Record Entries," *Journal of AHIMA* (March 2000).

BIBLIOGRAPHY

Abdelhak, Mervat, ed. *Health Information: Management of a Strategic Resource,* 2nd ed. Philadelphia: W.B. Saunders, 2001.

AHIMA. *Health Information Management Practice Standards: Tools for Assessing Your Organization.* Chicago: AHIMA, 1998.

Brandt, Mary. "Joint Commission Changes Authentication Requirements for Hospitals." *Journal of AHIMA* 67, no. 7 (July-August 1996): 32–33.

Clark, Jean. "Mastering the Information Management Standards." *Journal of AHIMA* 71, no. 2 (February 2000): 45–47.

Glondys, Barbara. *Documentation Requirements for the Acute Care Patient Record.* Chicago: AHIMA, 1999.

Halpert, Aviva M. "Access Audit Trails: En Route to Security." *Journal of AHIMA* 71, no. 8 (September 2000): 43–46.

Huffman, E. *Health Information Management,* 10th ed. Berwyn, Ill.: Physicians' Record Company, 1994.

Johnson, Thomas H., et al. "Reengineering Medical Records: The Dubois Regional Medical Center's Experience." *Journal of AHIMA* 69, no. 3 (March 1998): 57–59.

CHAPTER 6

Numbering and Filing Systems

Nancy Coffman-Kadish

E very HIM department maintains systems that identify each patient and his or her health record data, along with documentation of all the services provided to the patient. In addition, HIM systems provide for the ready retrieval of this information in whatever format it has been stored. More specifically, the efficient operation of the HIM department depends on effective systems and methods for performing the following functions:

- Merging and preserving the documentation of patient care provided by various professional services to an individual during an episode of care

- Merging or cross-referencing records of care that a patient receives during more than one episode of care

- Identifying each patient and his or her health record by a unique personal identification number (UPIN)

- Providing a designated filing location for each patient's health record

- Accounting for removal of any record from its filing location

The methods and systems that an HIM department uses to perform these functions depend on the types of patient care services provided, the annual number of admissions and visits, the computerized systems in place, and the department's budget and space allocation. A common goal among all HIM departments is to promote efficiency and accuracy in the maintenance of the health record and in the record identification and filing systems used to locate it. The role of the HIM professional is to evaluate the various methods and select the most efficient, cost-effective methods that allow the record to be quickly retrieved when needed. This chapter examines various record identification and filing systems commonly used in HIM departments.

RECORD IDENTIFICATION SYSTEMS

Currently, most health care facilities maintain health records in a paper-based format. Although some electronic medical record systems are nearly twenty years old, truly paperless records are rare today.[1] Most hospitals have paper-based records or some combination of paper-based and computer-based records. Therefore, this chapter primarily discusses the various methods available for identifying and filing paper records.

Alphabetical Filing

The easiest method of record identification is identifying the record by the patient's name. This method requires only the patient's name to file and retrieve the record—information that is attainable from the patient him- or herself. No separate system of cross-referencing the patient's name and health record number is needed. However, the accurate spelling of all patient names is of extreme importance. It is also important to create a system to track name changes, such as from marriage or divorce.

Although this system appears to be quite simple in that the information is obtainable from the patient and most people know how to alphabetize, it is not quite that easy to maintain. Different spellings of the same name (for example, Smith, Smithe, Smyth, Smythe, or Cindy, Cindi, Cyndi) and the complex spellings of some ethnic last names make an alphabetical filing system more difficult to accurately maintain than it would first appear. Therefore, it is important to thoroughly train staff to verify patient names and spelling and to accurately and consistently file alphabetically.

Another factor to consider with alphabetical record identification is patient confidentiality. Patient names are typically written on the file folder, which makes the name easily observable. In addition, because the record is not protected by identification numbers that would need to be obtained from another source, such as a number index or the MPI (see Chapter Seven), the record could be easily retrieved from the file by an unauthorized individual.

Alphabetical record identification systems are most appropriate for smaller health care offices or facilities with a stable population, such as a small solo physician or group practice office. It is also more practical for facilities with little or no computerization.

Numerical Identification

In any large system involving the names of individuals (such as bank accounts, charge accounts, life or health insurance policies, and so on), unique numbers are issued to differentiate one person from another. For health information systems, numbering methods typically include unit numbering, serial numbering, serial-unit numbering, annual numbering, numbering by Social Security number, family numbering, or numbering by another unique patient identification number. A numerical identification system for health records requires the use of a number index or master patient (or population) index (MPI) to cross-reference the patient's name with his or her assigned record number or numbers.

Unit Numbering System

A unit numbering system is based on the one-time issuance of a number to a patient. The same number is used to identify that patient and his or her health record on all subsequent admissions or visits. One unit numbering system can serve a number of functions within the health care facility. To provide rapid and accurate identification, the maintenance of an MPI using a computer system is desirable. At the time of patient registration, the admitting department can then obtain the health record number of any patient who has been previously registered in the system or can easily register a new patient. This unit number obtained via the MPI is used to identify patient health records, radiographic films, tracings, and the like. For patient accounting purposes, however, a separate account or billing number is usually assigned for each encounter.

Manual and Automated Issuance of Numbers. When a unit number is used, all departments issuing a number must be able to determine immediately whether a number already exists for an individual patient or whether a new number should be assigned. Provisions for issuing unit numbers can then be instituted as needed. If a manual system is used, a block of numbers is issued biweekly or monthly to each admitting area for use in initiating new health record numbers. In the more typical automated system, the computer program controls the issuance of numbers by automatically assigning the next sequential number to a new patient admission. Daily computer printouts of admissions and discharges are distributed from a data processing system. These lists contain the patient name and number, as well as institution-specific information. Many cross-checks can be performed with these admission, discharge, and transfer lists, including the verification of a patient unit number.

Procedures for Error Correction. The maintenance of either a manual or computer system requires documented procedures for handling errors that are inherent in number assignments. In a manual system, common clerical errors include the assignment of the same identification number to more than one patient, the transposition of digits in copying the identification number, and the assignment of a new identification number to a patient who already has one on file. In a computer system, the most common error is the assignment of a new number to a patient who already has a unit number. This last type of error is usually best corrected after the patient's discharge. When corrections are made in patient number assignments, all departments and services involved in the diagnostic workup and treatment of the patient should be notified of the change. The business office should also be notified. Steps for correcting errors in identification numbers should be carefully engineered to prevent mistakes and delays in the procedures for verification of patient identification, such as those used by radiographers and clinical laboratory sciences personnel.

Shelf Requirements for Records Filing. The use of a unit numbering system for the HIM department affects space allocations for filing records. Each shelf must accommodate growth in the size of individual records due to readmissions and ongoing visits to ambulatory care facilities. In assigning a given number of records to each shelf file, 25 percent of the shelf space should be set aside for future increases in the bulk of the records. Additional space will become available as records that are not used for three to five years are moved to the inactive file. However, in a unit numbering system usually only the unit number is reactivated and the health record remains in the inactive file.

The unit numbering system requires more intense service and control by the HIM department than do other numbering systems. However, it provides the basis for the integration of records for inpatient care, ambulatory care, emergency care, hospice care, long-term care, and home care.

Serial Numbering System

The serial numbering system is a method in which the patient receives a new record number for each inpatient admission or outpatient visit at the facility. In a facility that has a relatively stable patient population, such as a community hospital, one patient could have many numbers and therefore many health records filed in different locations. This method also requires the entry of each number into the manual MPI or maintenance in the computerized database.

A major advantage of this system is that it is easy to assign a number because it is not necessary to determine whether the patient has already been assigned a number. Major disadvantages are that it requires the maintenance of a number for each encounter, whether on an index card or in a computerized database. This requires a lot of valuable computer space. Also, higher supply costs are involved, as each encounter would require a new file folder for the new number. Serial numbering is much more time consuming when record retrieval is needed, as it is necessary to retrieve all the patient's records from multiple locations. Finally, the extra time required to locate a patient's entire record may discourage physicians from requesting "old records" because they don't want to wait for them, which may affect patient care negatively.

Serial-Unit Numbering System

The serial-unit numbering system assigns a new identification number to each patient and to his or her health record for each stay in the health care facility and for each episode of ambulatory, long-term, or emergency care. Each time a patient is seen, the previous records are brought forward and filed under the latest number issued. The serial-unit numbering system works best for health care facilities that do not have ambulatory or long-term care units. The constant movement of files in institutions with these units is inefficient.

The Serial-Unit System and the Unit Record. The serial-unit numbering system of filing is compatible with a unit record system for inpatient health records. Each time the patient is admitted, all previous inpatient records are brought forward and filed under the latest identification number that has been issued to the patient. The system requires a cross-referencing system for number identification in the MPI and in the file area. All serial identification numbers assigned to a particular patient are listed under his or her name in the MPI. As records are removed from their filing location, a cross-reference note to the latest identification is entered and documented in the old location. This is necessary in order to locate the records under the new number. In health care facilities with frequent readmissions, the health record number is continually updated, and the computer data are changed to designate the most recently assigned identification number. Health record files are continually guided to the current filing location.

Serial-Unit System and Ambulatory Care Programs. For health care facilities that provide ambulatory care services, the serial-unit numbering filing system is ineffective in integrating inpatient and outpatient health records. Ambulatory care records cannot be assigned new identification numbers on each visit without disrupting both patient care and the maintenance of an ongoing health record. When inpatient and outpatient health information systems are maintained separately, the identification numbers are cross-referenced at the time of the patient's admission to the health care facility. However, some means must be established to distinguish between the two numbering systems. Entering the year of registration in the ambulatory care program, followed by the serial registration number, is one means of differentiating the two numbering systems. Adding the year of registration in the identification number also makes it easy to spot records that are candidates for transfer from active to inactive files.

The continued use of the serial-unit numbering filing system in institutions with active ambulatory care programs should be assessed on the basis of the following questions:

- How successful is the system in achieving the goals of an integrated or unit health record system?

- How much time and expense is incurred in maintaining the serial-unit numbering system or two numbering systems?

- What is the percentage of error in misfiled data, and what is the impact of filing errors on patient care?

- What type of delays are being incurred because of a lack of reference to the most current identification number in various indexes and secondary files?

- What is the backlog in updating active files?

Annual Numbering System

Annual numbering, that is, serial-unit numbering that includes the last two digits of the current calendar year, may be used by facilities that serve a primarily transient population. In this system, the two digits representing the year are added to the end of a serial number. The year designation serves as a control number in retiring inactive records. In addition, the serial number, together with the calendar year, provides immediate data on the number of admissions or visits that occurred during a specific year.

Social Security Numbering System

Using Social Security numbers as patient identification numbers is not recommended. This system has been used by Veterans Administration hospitals, which receive assistance from the Social Security Administration for the location of unknown numbers. From the standpoint of logistics and personal privacy rights, however, the use of a Social Security number to identify both the patient and his or her health record should be discouraged. Numbering health records by the patient's Social Security number has various drawbacks, including these:

- The health care facility must control its patient identification numbering system, but it has no control over the Social Security number.

- The health care facility does not have access to Social Security Administration files to verify a patient's name and Social Security number. A non-Medicare patient could provide several different numbers, and the facility would have no way of verifying whether any of the numbers had actually been assigned to that individual by the Social Security Administration.

- The patient's Social Security number may not be available at the time of admission.

- The patient has the right to withhold his or her Social Security number without being denied care, creating the need for a separate numbering system or a pseudo–Social Security number. A dual numbering system must be maintained for such instances.

- A pseudo number could be disclosed in reports to third parties, who would assume that it was the patient's actual Social Security number.
- All number references would need to be updated when a patient's Social Security number is not available at the time of admission but becomes available later.
- Records or information about the patient could be easily identified with the patient's Social Security number and, therefore, could be exchanged, consolidated, and linked for purposes that may be unfair to the patient.

There is significant concern regarding the use of a standard, universal identification label such as a Social Security number. Confidentiality of the health record information is an important concern of the HIM professional. Systems must be put in place to protect health record information from unauthorized disclosure and patients from potential harm.

Family Numbering System

In another infrequently used numbering system, family medicine clinics may find it useful to identify individuals and their health records by family association. In a family numbering system, a unique number is assigned to each family, followed by a unique number to identify each member of the family. The family number is actually a household number, because it includes only individuals living within a given household. It includes grandparents, aunts, and uncles, for example, living in the same household, but it excludes family members who have moved away from the household. Therefore, the family number assignment may identify individuals who have different last names. The family numbering system is difficult to maintain because members of a household frequently change. Confidentiality of individual members' health data is also a concern.

Unique Health Identifiers

Over the past few years, much has been written about the creation of a unique patient-identifier numbering system to link records across the health care delivery system. The Administrative Simplification Provisions of the Health Insurance Portability and Accountability Act (HIPAA) require that the secretary of the U.S. Department Health and Human Services adopt standards for unique health identifiers (UHI) for individuals.[2] The key issues for the HIM profession with regard to the UHI include privacy, data integrity, and the accurate linkage of information. UHIs have been controversial because of the perception that all of an individual's information could be available through the unique identifier. Currently, UHIs for individuals are on hold until legislation is enacted specifically approving the standards and mechanisms in place to protect the individual.

FILING SYSTEMS

Paper health records are filed according to one of two systems: (1) an alphabetical system or (2) some form of numerical filing.

Alphabetical Filing

Records that use an alphabetical identifier must be filed with an alphabetical filing system. These records may simply be filed in strict alphabetical order—A to Z—by patient last name. For identical last names, the patient first name and then middle name are used to determine the filing order. When only the initial of the first name (or no middle name) is available, the rule of "nothing before something" is used. This means that an initial of "J" is filed before a name of "Julia." Each name is considered as a group for filing purposes. For example, last names with prefixes such as O', Mc, Van, and so on, are filed as if there were no apostrophe or space in the name. Hyphenated names are filed as if there were no hyphen.

Numerical Filing Systems

Although alphabetical filing is the simplest method to implement, facilities that have more than five thousand records, service transient populations, or have computerized systems typically assign numbers to identify their patients. If numerical identifiers are used, numerical filing is also used. Straight numerical and terminal digit (TD) are the two most commonly used systems.

Straight Numerical Filing System

The straight numerical filing system incorporates the sequential arrangement of records by health record identification numbers, starting with the lowest number and ending with the highest number. The highest numbers, which identify the most recent cases, represent the greatest amount of retrieval and filing activity. Therefore, most activity and personnel will be concentrated in one part of the file area.

Because this filing system does not evenly disperse the records or the activity and personnel for maximum use of the entire file area, one section can become congested when records are pulled for clinic appointments or loose reports are filed in the appropriate records. This results in the inefficient operation of the file area.

Personnel are usually familiar with the principle of filing by number sequence, so less training is needed. However, quality controls are needed to ensure that records are filed correctly. Unless the entire health record number is checked before the record is filed, it is possible to misfile it by a one-hundred- or a one-thousand-number sequence. Finding a misfile is usually more time consuming in a straight numerical sequence file than in a TD file; in those, colored folders may be used to enhance filing accuracy.

TD Filing

TD filing is a method that distributes health records equally in filing units throughout the file area. By providing for equal distribution, TD filing permits a more even workflow pattern. Personnel retrieve and file records in all parts of the file area rather than just one. The number is read from left to right for identification purposes and read from right to left for filing purposes.

The traditional TD method divides the patient number into three parts; newer methods divide the number into two parts. The traditional method identifies the last two digits of the health record number as the "primary or terminal digits," which identifies the first section of file location. For example, a file area is typically divided into 100 sections, starting with 00 and ending with 99. A health record number of 512640 would be read as 51–26–40, with the last two digits—40—designating the first section of the file location. All records ending in 40 would be located in a designated section. The second section of the filing arrangement is based on the middle two digits of the health record number—26. The health record 51–26–40 would be filed behind a shelf guide labeled "26–40," along with all other records that have the last four digits of 2640. If five second-order sections were allocated to each filing shelf, the TD arrangement and sequence of health records with the last four digits ranging from 2540 through 2940 could be filed as shown in the following example:

- Section one: 01–25–40, 02–25–40, 03–25–40, 04–25–40, 05–25–40, and so on

- Section two: 01–26–40, 02–26–40, 03–26–40, 04–26–40, 05–26–40, and so on

- Section three: 01–27–40, 02–27–40, 03–27–40, 04–27–40, 05–27–40, and so on

- Section four: 01–28–40, 02–28–40, 03–28–40, 09–28–40, 10–28–40, and so on

- Section five: 06–29–40, 07–29–40, 10–29–40, 11–29–40, 12–29–40, and so on

In the example, there are gaps in health record numbers behind the division for 28–40 and 29–40. These gaps represent records that have been moved to the inactive files. Removal of inactive records does not alter the TD filing arrangement.

The key to the TD system is a design that permits the file personnel to visualize the actual location of the record in the file when reading the health record number. The retrieval and filing time may be faster when the file clerk is able to read 51–26–40 as "Go to section 40, look behind guide 26, and retrieve (or file) record 51." In large health care facilities, the file room is divided into sections, with a file clerk responsible for each section. For example, section 1 covers records with numbers ending in 00–19; section 2 covers records with numbers ending in 20–39; section 3 covers records with numbers ending in 40 through 59, and so on.

Various shelving layouts should be considered to ensure maximal use of available file space. Typically, health records are sorted by health record number before filing into TD filing order with the use of bins or carts. When the record is returned to the permanent file area for filing, it is placed in the appropriate bin according to the last two digits of the patient number. For example, all records with numbers ending in 00 through 09 are placed in one bin; those ending in 10 through 19 in another bin, and so on. Sorting by number facilitates the filing task by separating the records according to the sections of the file area.

As mentioned earlier, other TD filing systems are in use. The 3TD system breaks the number into two sets of three digits. The last three numbers are considered the primary or terminal digits, and they determine the initial file location. The first three are then used to determine the filing order.

Training periods for file clerks learning to use the TD filing system often are slightly longer than for a straight numerical system. However, the advantages of the system compensate for the training time required.

Batch Filing Systems

A filing method commonly used for outpatient records is batch filing. Facilities that have large volumes of outpatient visits usually do not have the personnel available to file each outpatient visit record in the patient unit record. Not only does this require a lot of staff time but it results in voluminous records. Batch filing is a method whereby outpatient records are filed by the year of the visit and then in individual folders that indicate either the patient's last name or two or three digits of the patient number. Vendors have several different types of folders available.

Batch filing can be customized to meet the needs of the facility. The type of outpatient records placed in the batch file is determined by the individual facility. A facility may choose to place all outpatient records in the batch files or may choose to file outpatient surgery or emergency room records in the unit record and all others in the batch file. Reports filed in the batch files are then retrieved for patient care purposes or as otherwise requested.

Other Considerations in Filing Systems

Additional considerations in developing the health record filing system include record security, the choice between centralized and decentralized file areas, the numbering style, color coding system, and type of file folder to be used.

Security. Record security is of the utmost importance when developing a health record filing system. Records must be stored in a location that is secure to prevent unauthorized access. Records must be placed in a file or room that can be locked. The records must also be protected from hazards such as fire and water damage.

Centralized Versus Decentralized Files. A centralized file is one in which all records for a facility are in a single location. A centralized file area is convenient to maintain in a health care facility that has no satellite clinics. However, with the trend toward offering care off-site at a clinic or surgi-center of the main facility, the concept of decentralization is becoming commonplace. In decentralized filing, certain types of records are kept in different locations, typically where the record originated. For example, a hospital-owned oncology center may elect to house its own records and only forward a copy of the face sheet or summary sheet to the main hospital department for inclusion in the inpatient record.

With the decentralized record system, a procedure must be implemented to maintain the flow of information between the satellite facility and the main health care institution. The system ensures the indexing of the patient's ambulatory and inpatient care encounters, and the records for both types of visits are readily accessible. A fax machine can be used to transmit data to and from the decentralized sites. This, however, raises legal issues of confidentiality, authenticity, and validity of the document in the patient record. It is essential that the health care facility develop and maintain policies and procedures that define the types of information that may be faxed, and to whom and under what circumstances. AHIMA has published a practice brief titled "Facsimile Transmission of Health Information" to assist HIM professionals in the development of guidelines for the faxing of information.

Numbering Style. The method used to place the patient's identification number on forms, folders, and identification cards merits attention. It is common practice to divide identification numbers into groups of two or three digits, with a space or hyphen to accent the division. In some instances, a one-digit or two-digit division in a certain location within the number represents a code. As in the TD filing system, the last two digits indicate the filing section and the filing unit. Dividing a four-digit to six-digit number into a two-digit division (for example, 050785 would be written 05–07–85) promotes accuracy in reading and copying the number, as well as in filing the record.

A basic method that is used in some health care facilities is a three-part numbering style—that is, 00–00–00. This method provides uniformity, familiarity, and a basis for expansion. If this style were not in use and if the highest number in present use were a five-digit number (for example, 51234), the former numbers could easily be converted to a three-part style by adding a zero as the first digit (for example, 05–12–34). As mentioned earlier, six-digit numbers can also be grouped into two sets of three digits. Although a six-digit numbering system is the most common, these numbering methods may be used with a number as large as nine digits.

Color-Coding System. Health record folders are usually color coded to facilitate sorting and filing and to minimize misfiling problems. Color-coded folders were originally developed as part of TD filing systems. The color scheme on the folder is used to identify the file location for the health record number. Color coding may also be used with alphabetical filing systems in which the first few letters of the patient last name are color coded.

A color-coding system can be simple or detailed, depending on variables such as costs and the needs of the facility. Typically, color coding the numbers is kept simple, with no more than three or four of the health record numbers being placed on the file folder. Vendors offer many options in filing systems, such as preprinted color bars, pressure-sensitive color labels, laminated continuous strip labels, and the like.

Color-coding systems are also used by other departments. For example, radiology might color code film jackets to enhance filing accuracy or to indicate the latest date of the films within a jacket.

File Folders. There are many factors to consider when selecting appropriate file folders. The weight of the folder material should be selected, based on the length of time the record is kept in paper format and the activity of the file. Heavier weight should be used for records kept on paper for longer periods of time and for files in which there is heavy filing and retrieval activity. Reinforcement on the top and side panels is also important for these kinds of records. Folder bottoms should be scored to accommodate the facility's average size record. Folders are available with pouches on the front for microfiche, routing slips, or important reports that should be kept separate yet should remain within the contents of the folder.

The facility must also determine whether fasteners are to be placed in the folder to secure the record contents. Some facilities, such as physician offices, do not use fasteners because of the inconvenience they are thought to cause. However, fasteners are important to prevent the loss of reports. The size, location, and design style are also factors to consider.

Miscellaneous Patient Forms

The principle of centralizing all information pertaining to a patient in a single record is desirable, with a few exceptions. To provide a central filing location with easy access, patient-related correspondence and reports generated by outside parties are filed in the folder along with the patient's health record but are not considered a part of it. Such materials include patient-related correspondence from insurance carriers, government agencies, and other health care institutions. Summaries or reports of patient care that have been provided by another health care institution are filed with the patient's health record, but they are not considered to be a part of the health care facility record.

Chart Requisition and Tracking Systems

The selection of methods for requisitioning health records, charging out records, and tracking the location of records is just as important as the selection of numbering and filing systems and filing equipment. The HIM department is responsible for maintaining controls on records that are not in the files. Such methods may be computerized or manual, or a combination of the two.

Factors to be considered in developing or revising methods for requisitioning and charging out records include the following:

- *Identifying or instituting a uniform database for requisitioning and charging out records.* The database should include the health record number, the patient's name, the date of request, the date that the record was dispatched to the requester, the name of the person or ambulatory care center requesting the record, the name of the person calling for the record (if it is different from that of the person requesting it), and the location and telephone extension within the health care facility where the health record will be used and located.

- *Establishing a uniform size in a manual system (such as 3 × 5") for all requisition and charge-out forms.* In addition, paperwork can be simplified by designing multiple-part, carbonless forms. In this way, one copy can accompany the record, one can be placed in the charge-out file, and one can be placed in the outguide.

- *Developing policies to determine which staff members are and are not authorized to request records.*

- *Establishing a health record policy requiring that any record not in its filing location be accounted for.* This includes the records of patients who are currently being treated in the health care facility, records being completed, records being processed within the HIM department, and records being used for nondirect patient care purposes, such as quality management; all must be accounted for by an appropriate charge-out slip or entry into the computer system.

- *Ensuring the proper functioning of an automated system.* This includes ascertaining that the system accurately prioritizes software-generated requests, processes on-line inquiries from every system terminal, and tracks multiple volumes of the same record in multiple file-room locations.

With a few exceptions and some modification, the preceding considerations can be used in either a manual or computerized chart requisition and tracking system. In many departments, optical scanning equipment, such as bar codes and scanners, is used for documenting all record requests and returns. Many software packages that can track and locate records at any given time are available. Computer systems can generate requisition slips for outguides and "chart pull" lists that are based on pending requests for records. Programs also provide reports on record activity and staff workload. The HIM professional should review the available systems to select the most efficient one for the department's needs. A vast number of management and statistical reports are available via an automated system and should be reviewed by the appropriate department staff.

Bar coding is often used in HIM departments to track charts. Most health care institutions are using bar coding somewhere in the facility, such as in inventory tracking or patient identification. The machine-readable identification that is offered by bar-coding technology has many advantages over key entry. It can eliminate the need to reenter data, and it can drastically reduce the rate of error. Many computerized chart tracking systems use bar coding to sign records in and out of the HIM department

Health Information Management

and to facilitate on-line inquiries about the current locations of records. Bar coding may also be used to link paper records to electronic records.

IMPACT OF THE ELECTRONIC HEALTH RECORD

The implementation of the electronic health record will significantly affect all record systems involved with filing, chart tracking, and the like. The original definition of *computer-based patient record,* as it is defined in the Institute of Medicine study[3] of 1991, has evolved to reflect the changes in content, function, and structure of the health record. In 1999, this definition was revised to read as follows: "The electronic health record is defined as any information related to the past, present, or future physical or mental health or condition of an individual that resides in an electronic system(s) used to capture, transmit, receive, store, retrieve, link, and manipulate multimedia data for the primary purpose of providing health care and health-related services."[4] Whatever the definition, it is agreed that computerization of the patient record will revolutionize the basic functions of the HIM department. Although few hospitals today have a completely paperless health record, from the time of patient admission many aspects are computerized. The level of computerization affects all HIM department operations.

Currently, most administrative areas of a health care facility are already computerized. These areas include billing, financial management, ADT, health record abstracting, and the MPI. Many key clinical areas such as laboratory sciences, radiology, and pharmacy are also computerized; bedside terminals are available to capture nursing documentation. The health care institution's data network must meet the challenge of automating the exchange of the clinical and financial data while adhering strongly to the confidentiality of the health care data.

Chart requisition and tracking systems are nonexistent in a paperless environment. In their place are systems to allow authorized access to patient data and methods to monitor them. The electronic record allows concurrent access to multiple users. The space requirements for filing health records electronically are greatly reduced. Optical or laser disks are capable of storing more than 5 trillion (5,000,000,000,000) characters of data in an area of approximately 500 square feet. Paper records are stored on the optical disk and later retrieved for reproduction on high-resolution terminals. Images are reproduced by a laser printer to obtain a paper copy of the record.

Given the movement toward a paperless environment, the HIM professional must be involved in redesigning existing paper forms to allow the capture of data for scanning. However, the institution and HIM professional will also need to be prepared for potential problems; for example, it may not be possible to translate some of the data in the paper record into usable electronic data. As technology advances, the HIM professional will need to focus on efficient systems that reduce the amount of paper in the record while improving the quality of the information. Successful systems will not only store data effectively but will allow the information to be delivered efficiently to those who need it. Current and future technology thus will offer opportunities to improve both the efficiency of clinical information input and the effectiveness of clinical information output.

HEALTH INFORMATION MANAGEMENT IN MULTISITE SYSTEMS

Health record linkage in multisite health care systems is a concern of many HIM managers. Multihospital systems are commonplace, including integrated delivery systems (IDSs) that include multiple hospitals, long-term care, assisted living, primary care, ambulatory surgery, specialty clinics, and preventive medicine; the list goes on. Linkage between all or some of these sites is a requirement of many HIM departments. Although complex IDSs exist that include all of these services, health care systems that include only the main health care facility and one or more satellite ambulatory care centers or physician offices are more common.

Many innovative computerized health record systems have also been developed for ambulatory practice. Such systems provide an on-line display of clinical information and may be integrated to manage all aspects of the patient's encounter with a clinic, including scheduling, physician encounter, diagnosis, treatment, and billing. Developing a system for satellite facilities also enhances patient care by improving the availability, accessibility, timeliness, and organization of medical information.

Communications technology has significantly affected HIM in multisite facilities through the use of local area networks (LANs), wide area networks (WANs), and servers. In a LAN, multiple devices such as personal computers (PCs) are connected in a small geographic area. In a primary care clinic, ten PCs may be linked via a server to the health care facility's mainframe computer. This enhances communication between the satellite facilities and the main health care institution by allowing users to retrieve and use all data that are stored within the system. In a WAN, separate institutions may be linked. WANs are used for larger and more extensive environments that may be geographically distant from each other. A WAN creates a comprehensive information system that communicates clinical data among providers.

Traditionally, communication links between satellite clinics and health care facilities have allowed a clinic to gain access to data in the central facility's mainframe system or database. LANs and WANs allow expanded communication among the various facilities, as well as with pharmacies, third-party payers, and clinical laboratories. In using a networked system, reports from the laboratory, radiology, and other departments (such as operative and consultation reports) are automatically transmitted to PCs or fax machines located at the satellite centers. Linkage with third-party payers is accomplished for the precertification of procedures or admissions, claims status inquiries, electronic claims, and eligibility requests. Automatic results reporting for clinical laboratory tests is accomplished through the network as well. The result is improved efficiency for both the satellite clinic and the central health care facility.

The HIM professional working in the development of the computerized health information system for the satellite facility must also be involved in the significant confidentiality issues. Access to patient data is regulated because physicians, nurses, paramedical personnel, and other support staff need to have access to the clinical data at different times. Each unit of the health care organization has specific requirements, but all users should be properly trained to ensure that record confidentiality is maintained. As computer-based satellite record systems continue to evolve, the HIM professional will play a significant role in that evolution and in the protection of health records from unauthorized use.

CONCLUSION

The HIM professional has responsibility for maintaining numbering and filing systems that make the patient health record available at all times to authorized users. The department may use a variety of the systems described in this chapter, with the end result being an efficient and effective method of retrieving information.

The extent of computerization affects the efficiency and speed of the retrieval. Factors such as size of the facility, volume of patients seen, and number of the satellite facilities all have an impact on the record systems selected. Whatever the system, it needs to merge, preserve, and provide thereafter the documentation of patient care rendered by various professionals during an episode of care.

REFERENCES

1. M. Hagland, "Moving Gradually Toward a Paperless World." *Journal of AHIMA* 71, no. 8 (September 2000): 26–31.
2. B. Cassidy, "HIPAA: Understanding the Requirements." *Journal of AHIMA* 71, no. 4 (April 2000).
3. R. S. Dick and E. B. Steen, eds., "The Computer-Based Patient Record: An Essential Technology for Health Care." Washington, D.C.: National Academy Press, 1991.
4. G. Murphy, et al. *Electronic Health Records: Changing the Vision.* Philadelphia: W.B. Saunders, 1999.

BIBLIOGRAPHY

Abdelhak, Mervat, ed. *Health Information: Management of a Strategic Resource,* 2nd ed. Philadelphia: W.B. Saunders, 2001.

Cofer, J., et al. *Information Management: The Compliance Guide to the Joint Commission Standards,* 2nd ed. Marblehead, Mass.: Opus Communications, 2000.

DeLuca, J., et al. *The CEO's Guide for Health Care Information Systems.* San Francisco: Jossey-Bass, 2001.

CHAPTER 7

Secondary Health Data

Nancy Coffman-Kadish

Health care facilities maintain many different secondary health data sets. These indexes, databases, and registers are used to classify and locate health records and other health information. Ease in locating information facilitates patient-care management and research, quality-of-care review, utilization management, and administrative and financial functions, as well as compliance with federal and state regulations and licensure requirements.

Due to technological advances in computer systems and an ever-increasing demand for information, most indexes, databases, and registers used in health care are now computerized. Thus the emphasis in this chapter is on computerized systems. However, because some older systems are still in use, manual procedures are briefly discussed as well.

NUMBER INDEX

In order to ensure that each patient is assigned a unique health record number, health care institutions maintain a number index. Any errors in health record numbers or duplication of numbers must be immediately corrected. This important log is a numerical listing of health record numbers with the name of the patient to whom each number is assigned. The purpose of the number index is to ensure that two or more patients have not been assigned the same health record number. If there is a question about a number, the number index is the reference that is consulted. To function as a reliable reference, the number index must be a complete and accurate listing of each number issued.

The number index may be maintained in either a manual or computerized format. In a manual format, the number index may be as simple as a handwritten numerical listing, with the patient numbers in one column and the name of the patient to whom each number is assigned in the other. In facilities where the computer system does not automatically maintain the number index through the MPI but a PC is available, the HIM professional may keep the number index in a spreadsheet program. An advantage of using this method is that the program can also do an alphabetical sort to maintain both a number index and a cross-referenced alphabetical index.

If the health care facility's computer system automatically assigns numbers to patient health records, a separate number index does not need to be maintained. In this instance, careful monitoring of the accuracy of the MPI is essential to ensure that there are no errors or duplications in the assignment of patient numbers.

MASTER PATIENT INDEX

The master patient index, also known as the master population or person index, or MPI, is a file that identifies all patients who have been admitted or treated by a health care institution. All patients registered to receive care as either inpatients or outpatients, including referral, clinical, emergency care, home care, or other care provided by the facility, are listed individually in the MPI. As the key to locating patient records, whether in paper or electronic format, a complete and accurate MPI is a crucial part of an institution's patient information system. The MPI identifies all patients who have been treated in the health care facility or enterprise, as well as the health record number associated with the name.

In this age of integrated health care delivery systems, maintenance of an accurate MPI is more important than ever. The MPI is a crucial informational link in the development of community health information networks, the establishment of multihospital systems, and the vertical integration of hospitals, physician practices, home care agencies, and long-term care and other non-acute care facilities. In these environments, it is particularly important to facilitate mergers of various indexes to create an enterprisewide MPI that provides access to longitudinal patient records. The longitudinal record includes all health and illness data collected on an individual from birth until death. The end result of data mergers should be an accurate and effective MPI that links the patient to facilities within an organization or enterprise and across patient care settings.

Although the MPI is usually computerized, some institutions still use a manual system consisting of file cards ($2^1/_4 \times 3"$ or $3 \times 5"$) housed in a cabinet or electrically powered file. Whether computer-based or manual, the MPI should contain sufficient information to readily identify a patient and his or her health record number. In either format, the MPI should be maintained permanently.

Minimum Data Elements

Two levels of data elements should be included in the MPI: (1) demographic data and (2) visit-level data. The MPI should contain sufficient demographic data to easily identify the patient and his or her file. The demographic data contain identifying information about the patient and usually do not change from visit to visit. However, it is recommended that these data be verified during registration for each visit and updated as needed. The visit-level data include information that changes with each encounter. The American Health Information Management Association (AHIMA) suggests that the minimum data set for patient identification in the MPI include the following information:[1]

Demographic Level

- Internal patient identification—health record number
- Person name—last name, first name, and middle name or initial, name suffixes and prefixes
- Date of birth—birth date by month, day, and four-digit year
- Date-of-birth qualifier to indicate whether the date of birth is actual or an estimate
- Gender
- Race
- Ethnicity
- Address by street, city, state, and ZIP code
- Alias or previous name
- Social Security number
- Facility identification
- Universal patient identifier (when established)

Visit Level

- Account number
- Admission or encounter date
- Discharge or departure date
- Encounter or service type
- Patient disposition

These data elements should be accurately matched with persons being registered to minimize duplicate records within a facility and across patient care settings.

Optional data elements that may also be maintained in the MPI include those in the following list:

Health Information Management

- Marital status
- Telephone number
- Mother's maiden name
- Place of birth
- Advance directive and surrogate decision-making information
- Organ donor status
- Emergency contact
- Allergies or reactions
- Problem list

Because it is costly to enter and store data, whether the system is paper- or computer-based, an institution should only keep information that it will use. Provision should made for the correction of errors in a name or date of birth, for cross-referencing name changes, such as a change in a woman's surname upon marriage, and for the use of hyphenated names.

The MPI, long the key to numerically filed paper-based records, is now also the key to electronic data repositories and integration of all information across the continuum of care. Thus the data in the MPI must be organized in such a way that it is complete and accurate and is maintained in a manner that ensures the protection of patient privacy.

Filing Systems

The filing arrangement within the MPI usually follows one of two systems: (1) alphabetical or (2) phonetic. In the alphabetical system, patients' names are filed in strict alphabetical order by last name, with secondary alphabetical filing by first name, as in the following example:

Johansen, David

Johanssen, Alexander

Johanssen, Andrew

Johnson, George

Johnson, Julia

The phonetic system, which may be preferred by health care facilities that serve ethnically diverse communities, is better known by the trade name Soundex—a product originated by Remington-Rand Office Systems. The phonetic filing system is based on retaining the first letter of the last name as the first order of filing and then translating the next three types of consonants into a three-digit code. Examples of names in a phonetic filing system are found in Table 7.1.

Table 7.1. Examples of Names in a Phonetic Filing System

Code Assignment

Name	First File Order	Secondary File Order
Agee, Deloris	A-200	Deloris
Aigew, Doris	A-200	Doris
Agew, Doris	A-200	Doris
Bissenger, Olga	B-252	Olga
Basengelman, Olga	B-252	Olga
Johanssen, Richard	J-525	Richard
Johnson, Richard	J-525	Richard
Janssen, Robert	J-525	Robert
Olsen, Erik	O-425	Erik
Olson, Erik	O-425	Erik
Orlee, Claude	O-640	Claude
Quackenbush, Jacob	Q-251	Jacob
Quandt, Ella	Q-530	Ella
Quant, Ella	Q-530	Ella
Sanchez, Jaimee	S-520	Jaimee
Sanchoz, James	S-520	James

Last name, first name, and birth date usually suffice for the ready identification of most patients when the phonetic filing system is used. Variations of the phonetic filing system have been developed for use in computerized patient indexes, pharmacy or drug formulary indexes, and other name-based indexes.

Quality Control

The HIM professional is responsible for the quality of the MPI, regardless of whether a computerized or a manual system is used. Quality control measures include auditing patient identification data for spelling, completing the entry of required data, and checking for filing order and duplications. In addition, personnel in both the admitting department and the HIM department must be made aware of their important role in maintaining data accuracy and completeness at the time the data are entered into the MPI.

Whether computerized or manual, the MPI must be monitored for its accuracy and adherence to minimum data requirements. For example, if an error is made in the spelling of a name as it is entered into the system, it is extremely difficult to subsequently find or enter information on that patient.

Duplication in health record numbers is a special problem that can be caused by incomplete patient demographic information, errors in previous entries, or failure to carefully check for an existing MPI file when registering patients for subsequent visits. The institution should have written procedures for handling any duplication in health record number assignments. When duplication errors are discovered, new numbers must be issued to all but one of the patients, and corrections must be made throughout the health information system.

When a computerized MPI is used, individual files can be accessed and reviewed. The data are sorted by using various computer programs, and the accuracy of the demographic information can be checked, along with other edits such as admission and discharge dates, age, and health record number duplication. Misfiling errors cannot occur in a computerized system, which is relatively error-free if correct information is entered initially. However, it is important to remember that patient confidentiality is a salient issue with the computerized MPI, because computer terminals available throughout the facility make information accessible to all departments. The facility must devote the necessary resources to integrate and support a computerized MPI that consistently and correctly identifies patients while it protects their privacy.

Patient privacy is perhaps more easily maintained with a manual MPI system. However, because misfiling errors can occur, it is essential to check the filing performed by each person who enters information into the system.

The MPI is the key to the retrieval of health records for patient care purposes. It also contains the demographic items that, once entered into a computerized health information system, provide the core data for use in studies of patient accounts. These demographic items also are used in statistical studies of case-mix (the categories of patients, including both type and volume, that are treated by a facility).

Back-Up Measures

It is important to have back-up measures in place for automated MPIs in case of computer downtime. One option is to have a computer that is off-line to the facility's main system and in which the MPI data are backed up each night. Other options include paper printouts, computer output microfiche (COM), or computer output to laser disk (COLD) that should be routinely generated and available for staff use in record retrieval.

DISEASE AND OPERATION INDEXES OR DATABASES

The disease and operation index or database is a compendium of information, arranged by diagnosis and procedure, that provides, at a minimum, health record numbers of patients in which information on specific illnesses, injuries, or procedures can be found. The disease and operation indexes may take the form of reports generated from the clinical database or a manual system maintained in a card file. In either instance, it is a list of all cases in disease code order and procedure code order. This database is a cross-referencing tool for locating health records by diagnosis or procedure to carry out activities related to the following:

- Epidemiological and biomedical studies

- Health services research studies

- Statistical data on occurrence rates, age, sex, and complications or associated conditions

- Continuous quality improvement (CQI) and total quality management (TQM) activities

- Consultation on patient response to treatment in previous cases for applicability in a current case

- Review of health records for compliance with accreditation standards, licensing standards, and regulatory requirements for adequacy of documentation

- Continuing medical education

To ensure that every inpatient health record is accounted for in the disease and operation indexes, only authorized personnel should have access to the database, and only those persons who have been trained to check the accuracy of data entered from a source document should enter data.

Because CQI activities address outpatient and emergency care, provision must be made for retrieving outpatient and emergency records by diagnoses, either by establishing a separate database for outpatient and emergency records or by merging such records with the existing inpatient clinical database.

Required Information

The number of data items included in the disease and operation indexes depends on the needs of the individual health care institution. However, basic data for any type of disease and procedure index should include the following items:

- The illness, injury, and procedure classification code
- The patient's health record number
- The sex and age of the patient
- The identification of the responsible physician by code or name
- The dates of admission and discharge or the year of hospitalization and length of stay in days
- Any outcome of death and the findings from a subsequent autopsy
- Any additional disease or procedure codes

The disease and procedures indexes are commonly computerized through an in-house computer system or a commercial discharge data service. Some state hospital associations and third-party payers also process discharge data on a per-discharge basis. The Uniform Hospital Discharge Data Set (UHDDS), in use since the 1970s, contains the minimum core requirements related to the collection of individual hospital discharge data for Medicare and Medicaid patients. Among the items that institutions must record for each patient are the principal diagnosis, other diagnoses, the principal procedure, and other significant procedures. It is essential that all such information be recorded accurately.

When the disease and procedure indexes are the products of a multipurpose discharge abstracting system, more data are available as needed through computer printouts. When manual indexes are maintained, the number of data items is kept to the minimum needed for record-retrieval purposes. It is not cost-efficient to enter nonessential data.

Computerized Format

In almost all health care institutions, some type of computerized database system exists, of which the disease and operation indexes are a part. The facility may choose to periodically generate disease and operation index printouts in coded form (ICD-9-CM[2] for inpatient diagnoses and procedures and Current Procedural Terminology[3] [CPT] for some outpatient procedures). However, due to the volume of the reports and data gener-

Health Information Management

ated, most HIM departments choose to retrieve data on an as-needed basis. The database software allows the HIM professional to write ad hoc reports to retrieve clinical information, including only the specific diagnosis or procedure codes, time period, patient age, disposition, and so on needed for individual CQI studies or other types of requests.

In addition to the indexes previously described, many multihospital systems, state hospital organizations, and outside commercial services can provide comparative reports on system, local, state, and national statistics. Such statistics detail, in part, length-of-stay overall, diagnosis or diagnosis related groups (DRGs), percentage of occupancy, and morbidity and mortality rates. The data can be sorted by source, physician, and unit, or by a variety of demographic items. The ability to classify information in different ways facilitates the quality improvement process. This permits a facility to set a benchmark for its performance in comparison to those of other organizations.

Physician Index

The physician index lists doctors by name or unique personal identification number (UPIN), thus providing the health record numbers of patients who received treatment or consultation from a particular physician. As with the disease and operation indexes, the physician index may be maintained either manually or electronically. If manual, the index is maintained with a card file, filed either alphabetically by physician name or in numerical order by physician identification number. Usually, data entered into a manual system are limited to avoid unnecessary work. The data elements entered into a physician index may include the patient's health record number, the patient's age and sex, the date of admission, the length-of-stay in days, the disposition, and any surgical procedures performed. Consultation entries usually contain the patient's health record number, the date of admission, and identification of the entry as a consultation provided to another physician's patient. However, most physician indexes are a product of the facility's clinical database, and retrieval is performed on an as-needed basis, setting necessary parameters for an ad hoc report.

Uses of the Index

An important use of data from the physician index is the tabulation of data in physician-coded form to determine patient admission and length-of-stay rates for individual physicians. Such data are used in physician reappointments, utilization management studies throughout the health care facility, and CQI activities. An individual physician may also use the data when applying for board certification in his or her specialty.

With a computerized clinical database system, case-mix data relative to an individual physician are also available. The retrieval of such data often is tied to economic credentialing—that is, reviewing a physician's cost-efficiency on the basis of the DRG and using these data to make credentialing and reappointment decisions at the health care facility. Only the health care facility's CEO, usually in cooperation with the executive committee or the chief of the medical staff, can authorize access to this information by other persons or the disclosure of data in physician-identifiable form.

Data Quality and Security

When the physician index is generated by a facility's computerized health information system, data quality and data security are key concepts. The HIM professional should focus on maintaining the necessary information, ensuring that it is correct, and preventing unauthorized access to these very confidential data.

Because the physician index is regarded as a confidential record, access to it must be limited to authorized persons. Every physician listed in the index has the right to access the data that pertain to him or her. The health care facility's governing board and CEO have the right to access in accordance with their duties and responsibilities for ensuring the quality of patient care and conducting business affairs. The credentials committee of the organized medical staff has the right to access as it relates to staff reappointment and reappraisal of privilege delineation.

Index of Diagnoses

Ambulatory care facilities with family medicine or primary care programs may have an interest in maintaining a specialized statistical data system that involves an index of diagnoses referenced to patients' health record numbers. The data items collected relate to the services provided, treatments given, findings or diagnoses, and professional staff directly involved in providing the care and services. Diagnoses are coded using the ICD-9-CM classification system and procedures using the CPT system. Computerization allows for data display by physician, payer, service, principal diagnosis, principal procedure, and so on.

REGISTERS MAINTAINED BY HEALTH CARE FACILITIES

Health care institutions may also maintain a variety of registers. The need to maintain certain types of registers can be determined by the requirements for record control measures or by state regulations imposed on the facility. Computerized health information systems allow for maintaining all registers through the on-line system. Manual systems then are not needed. If a computerized system is not available, these registers are typically maintained in log books.

Patient Register

The patient register (sometimes known as the admission register) is a chronological list of patients' names arranged by date of inpatient admission. Minimum data items required are the date of admission, the patient's name, and the health record number. Additional items often include room assignment, sex, and the name of the attending physician. A copy of the daily list of admissions and births generated by the facility's admission, discharge, and transfer (ADT) system serves as an admission register. State licensing laws often include requirements for a patient registration log or an admission register. Computerized HIM systems can easily generate such reports.

Birth and Death Registers

Health care institutions also maintain birth and death registers. Many state vital records laws require the maintenance of birth and death registers. These registers may be maintained as a part of the health care facility's information system's database or as a log that is kept manually. AHIMA recommends that facilities maintain birth and death registers permanently.[4]

A birth register is a listing of all births at the facility. The purpose of the register is to be able to re-create a birth certificate if necessary. The register may be maintained in the delivery, or obstetrical, department or in the HIM department. The department responsible for completing birth certificates is also responsible for maintaining the birth register. The register information can be simple or detailed, depending on the needs of the obstetrical service and the health care facility. Minimum data include the date and time of birth, the sex of the baby, the status of the baby (live birth or fetal death), the name of the mother, the name of the physician or staff member in attendance at the time of delivery, and the date that the birth certificate was forwarded to the local registrar of vital records.

A death register—a chronological list of all patients who expired in the facility or who were dead on arrival—may be maintained in the HIM department or in the pathology or admitting department. A computerized register, also a part of the institution's health information system, contains the date of death, the name of the physician who completed the medical portion of the death certificate, and the name of the funeral director, coroner, or medical examiner who removed the body from the health care facility. The funeral director typically is responsible for completing the remainder of the death certificate and filing it with the local registrar of vital records. When the body is removed by the coroner or medical examiner for examination, the cause-of-death portion of the death certificate is completed by that official. The health care facility obtains a receipt for the body from the party that removes it. This receipt may be filed either in the patient's health record or in the department of pathology.

Operating Room Register

The operating room register is a list of all operative procedures performed in a facility's department of surgery. Typically computer-based, the register includes the date of each operation, the patient's name and health record number, and the names of the surgeons and assistants. The register provides statistical data for a variety of purposes within the institution, such as utilization management, case-load analysis, and CQI activities. In some states, the register is required by law. AHIMA recommends that the register of surgical procedures be maintained permanently.[5]

Emergency Department Register

Patients who are treated in the emergency department are listed in a chronological register that is maintained in the emergency department or service. The Joint Commission accreditation standards require that a control register shall be maintained on every patient seeking emergency or urgent care. This control register may include the following information for individuals seeking care: identification (such as name, age, and sex), date, time, means of arrival, nature of complaint, disposition, and time of departure. Patients who are dead on arrival are typically entered into the emergency department register; however, a health record is not generated.

Statistical data can be compiled from the emergency department register and used for monthly reports. They can also be used in case-mix analysis or in studies of utilization management, quality assessment, and risk identification. The computerization of data in the department facilitates all clinical data management activities.

Special Registries

In addition to the databases, indexes, and registers already described, health care facilities may maintain a variety of other special subject indexes. For example, institutions with a burn center may wish to maintain an index that provides specific statistical data on the treatment provided and on the utilization of the specialized service. Or a facility treating patients with AIDS-HIV may develop a special registry for research purposes. Before such registers are created, the cost of maintaining the database should be justified on the basis of interest in and actual use of the data and on the basis of requirements for participation in payment programs.

Cancer Registry. Typically, a health care institution's cancer program consists of four components: (1) the cancer committee, (2) the clinical program and cancer conferences, (3) patient care evaluation, and (4) management of the cancer database. The cancer registry is a system designed for the collection, management, and analysis of data on persons with diagnoses of cancer. The major purposes of the registry are to provide lifetime follow-up of the cancer patient and to provide meaningful information for research, statistics, and CQI activities. The patient's health record is the basic source document from which pertinent information is abstracted for use in the registry.

The responsibility for maintaining the cancer registry is usually assigned to the cancer registrar. This individual may be an HIM professional who is a registered health information administrator (RHIA) or a registered health information technician (RHIT); or the individual may be a certified tumor registrar (CTR)—a professional who has successfully completed the certification examination of the National Tumor Registrar Association.

Cancer registrars are guided by the publications of the Commission on Cancer (COC) of the American College of Surgeons: the *Cancer Program Standards*[6] and the *Registry Operations and Data Management (ROADS).*[7] These publications outline requirements for health care facilities concerning the quality of all oncology care provided to cancer patients. Two quality care improvement or enhancement activities must be documented each year, and the registry must submit data to the National Cancer Data Base (NCDB).[8] It is anticipated that *ROADS* will be replaced with the Facility Oncology Registry Data Standards (FORDS) in the future.

In meeting the requirements just outlined, the cancer registrar's responsibilities include abstracting data, maintaining an index of patients' names and addresses for follow-up studies on the outcome of the malignancy, and maintaining a statistical index cross-referenced to the patients' health records regarding the type and site of the malignancy and patients' records of history and treatment, when applicable. With an on-line computer system, the cancer registry and all its component parts are typically maintained electronically. Computerized abstracting has many advantages over previous manual systems, and the follow-up function is much easier to operate. For example, computerized follow-up letters and statistical tables are easily generated using one of the many cancer registry software programs currently available.

The COC grants approval of cancer registry programs in health care facilities based on compliance with ACS guidelines. In many states, the cancer registry program is carried out at the state level, and health care facilities must submit abstract data from patients' health records. If a statewide registry is in existence, the HIM professional must plan staffing adequate to perform the required functions.

The National Program of Cancer Registries has been implemented by the Centers for Disease Control and Prevention (CDC) to provide funding for states to improve existing cancer registries and to set standards for completeness, timeliness, and quality of cancer registry data. HIM professionals must know the specific reporting requirements in their state regarding cancer registries and what their facility must do to meet legislative requirements.

Trauma Registry. A trauma registry may be established to track the outcome of care for serious trauma patients who are treated at the health care facility or trauma center. A sophisticated registry can maintain various data elements and also be used to monitor quality, design prevention programs, and conduct research. The information maintained in trauma registries around the country is not standardized. However, data elements typically include the following areas:

- Demographics

- Injury information (time, place, date)

- Information gathered by the emergency medical service provider

- Referring health care facility

- Emergency department admission information

- Emergency department treatment

- Health care facility diagnoses and procedures

- Severity measurements

- Probability of survival

- Quality assessment indicators

- Complications

- Outcome

As computer-based patient records become the norm, opportunities will exist for the automatic linking of the trauma registries to the CPR. Demographic and other information will be downloaded from a facility's mainframe instead of being reentered, as is now being done.[9]

Organ Transplant Registry and Other Specialized Registries. In an organ transplant registry, an index may be maintained to identify the organs or tissues removed from brain-dead patients for transplantation purposes. The index identifies such items as the patient's health record number, the organ(s) or tissue removed, the date of the procedure, and identification of any outside team that performed the procedure. This "harvesting" of organs for transplantation purposes can also be coded using an appropriate code from the Current Procedural Terminology (CPT) system. In health care facilities that have transplantation programs, the HIM department links the recipient's health record number to the donor's entry.

Special indexes or registers can also be established to meet the needs of an individual or group of staff physicians or a specialized community need. Examples include a database for birth defects, diabetes, or implants.

These may be needed only for a specific time period, so steps should be taken annually to determine whether each special index is needed and is still being used.

CONCLUSION

Secondary health data are key information sources within the HIM department. The HIM professional must use current systems for the maintenance of these indexes, registers, and registries and strive to ensure that they are accurate and complete at all times. An accurate and complete primary patient record facilitates correct entry of those data into the computer database, with the end result being reliable data for the facility. The HIM professional's skills in research, computer data query, and statistical reporting are integral to efficient data storage and display. By using a common database to collect and integrate systems used in all indexes, registers, and registries, the health care facility can develop and implement strategies that affect the quality of care, the cost of care, and the efficiency with which care is provided.

REFERENCES

1. AHIMA, Practice Brief, "Master Patient (Person) Index (MPI): Recommended Core Data Elements," *Journal of AHIMA* (July 1997).
2. Health Care Financing Administration, *International Classification of Diseases*, 9th rev., *Clinical Modification* (Washington, D.C.: Department of Health and Human Services, Public Service, 2002).
3. American Medical Association, *Current Procedural Terminology* (Chicago: AMA, 2002).
4. AHIMA, Practice Brief, "Retention of Health Records," *Journal of* AHIMA (June 1999).
5. Ibid.
6. American College of Surgeons, *Standards of the Commission on Cancer. Volume I: Cancer Program Standards* (Chicago: ACS, 1996): 9–59.
7. American College of Surgeons, *Standards of the Commission on Cancer. Volume II: Registry Operations and Data Standards (ROADS)* (Chicago: ACS, 1996): 29–34.

8. Sue Watkins, "Managing Clinical Data: A Cancer Registries Update," *Journal of AHIMA* 68, no. 7 (July-August 1997): 22–25.
9. Elizabeth Garthe, "Overview of Trauma Registries in the United States," *Journal of AHIMA* 68, no. 7 (July-August 1997): 26–31.

BIBLIOGRAPHY

Abdelhak, Mervat, et al. *Health Information: Management of a Strategic Resource.* Philadelphia: W.B. Saunders, 2001.

Huffman, E. *Health Information Management,* 10th ed. Berwyn, Ill.: Physicians' Record Company, 1994.

Koch, G. *Basic Allied Health Statistics and Analysis,* 2nd ed. Canada: Delmar, 2000.

Koering, S. "A Cancer Program's Seal of Approval," *Journal of AHIMA* 73, no. 1 (January 2002): 40–44.

Watkins, S. "Cancer Registries," *Topics in Health Information Management* 17, no. 3 (February 1997).

CHAPTER 8

Coding, Compliance, and Reimbursement

Elizabeth A. Contant

Coding and analyzing data are key operations of a health care organization. The transformation of quality health care data into meaningful health care information is necessary to assess the quality of patient care and to improve its effectiveness. The quality of health care depends, in large part, on the quality of health care information. Thus clinical data quality is and will continue to be a top priority for health care organizations.

Before 1983, the codes recorded by department personnel were used to generate statistics and to form the basis for various indexes maintained by the department, such as the disease and procedure indexes (described in Chapter Six). Since the advent of DRGs and the prospective payment system (PPS) in 1983, reimbursement for care rendered by the health care facility has been determined by the codes and the DRGs into which patients are classified. In addition, since 1966 reimbursement to clinics and physician offices has been determined by the CPT codes submitted for each service. The financial strength of these institutions is largely determined by their ability to develop accurate and efficient billing processes and to recognize the need for knowledgeable and credentialed coders to optimize reimbursement.

Linking the coding and classification system to reimbursement has been an efficient means for communicating health care information between providers and carriers. However, it has also brought to the forefront the need for accurately coded data and compliance with coding guidelines. Many carriers, particularly Medicare, now closely scrutinize billing claims to ensure compliance with coding guidelines and health care laws. The accurate coding of data is a critical requirement for all health care facilities.

The coding and classification systems currently used in health care range from those that are statistical in nature to others that represent a catalog of terms for describing and recording clinical, pathological, or procedural terms. This chapter examines the two coding and classification systems that predominate in health care billing, reimbursement, and database systems: (1) the *International Classification of Diseases, 9 Revision, Clinical Modification*[1] (ICD-9-CM) and (2) the Physicians' *Current Procedural Terminology*[2] (CPT). Because HIM professionals should be familiar with the existence and purpose of other classification systems designed for use in the health care field, this chapter examines a few of these systems.

DEFINITION OF KEY ABBREVIATIONS

Many abbreviations that are used in the coding industry warrant definition. Individuals who work with clinical coding and classification systems should be familiar with the following abbreviations:

APC (ambulatory payment classification): A case-mix system for federal reimbursement of ambulatory care services. Services are grouped by similarities in clinical and resource utilization.

CCA (certified coding associate): An individual who has successfully passed the entry-level coding credentialing examination administered by AHIMA.

CCS (certified coding specialist): An individual who has successfully passed the facility-based coding credentialing examination, which is administered by AHIMA.

CCS-P (certified coding specialist–physician-based): An individual who has successfully passed the physician-based credentialing examination administered by AHIMA.

DRG (diagnosis related group): A case-mix system that places patients into related groups; the group determines reimbursement for hospitalized patients with health care coverage under Medicare.

CMS (Centers for Medicare and Medicaid Services), formerly known as HCFA (Health Care Financing Administration): An agency of the U.S. government responsible for the Medicare program and the federal government's role in the Medicaid programs. The agency established the Conditions of Participation with which providers must demonstrate compliance to be eligible for Medicare and Medicaid reimbursement.

HCPCS (HCFA's Common Procedure Coding System): A uniform method for health care providers and medical suppliers to report professional services, procedures, and supplies.

PPS (prospective payment system): A payment method in which the amount of the payment is fixed in advance of the services rendered; the rate is established annually by the government.

RBRVS (Resource-Based Relative Value Scale): A schedule system used for reimbursement of physician services.

INTERNATIONAL CLASSIFICATION OF DISEASES— ICD-9-CM

The HIPAA Final Rule has designated ICD-9-CM as one of the approved code sets for reporting diagnoses and inpatient procedures. The Final Rule also requires the use of ICD-9-CM by most health plans by October 16, 2002.[3]

The International Classification of Diseases is a classification system developed by the World Health Organization (WHO). Revisions are made yearly, and major new editions are published every ten to fifteen years. The ninth edition, published by the WHO in 1993, is currently in use in the United States and contains the most significant changes in the history of the ICD. ICD-10 has been implemented in many countries, including the United States, for mortality reporting. A date has not been set for the implementation of ICD-10-CM for diagnosis reporting in the United States. The tenth edition will be more specific in the reporting of disease information. Each area of clinical specialization will include codes for greater specificity and newly recognized conditions. Other modifications to ICD-10 include the addition of sixth digits, combining underlying condition (dagger) codes with manifestation (asterisk) codes, and new combination codes for diagnoses and symptoms.[4]

A drawback of the current ICD-9-CM is that it does not incorporate standard definitions, which results in inaccurate and inconsistent data and difficult data retrieval. ICD-10-CM will correct this deficiency by incorporating standard definitions. The ICD-10-Procedure Coding System (ICD-10-PCS) will also replace the procedure section of ICD-9-CM. This procedural classification system, currently under development and testing, will be more complete, expandable, and multiaxial and will be able to incorporate standardized terminology. It will use a seven-character, alphanumeric code structure, divided into sections according to the type of procedure (medical, surgical, imaging). The first character will specify the section, and the remaining characters (2–7) will describe the type of procedure, the body part, and additional information.[5] When complete, both ICD-10 systems will enhance the ability of health information coders to determine accurate codes. Accurate and complete coded data must be available in all health care settings to improve the quality and effectiveness of patient care, ensure appropriate reimbursement, and permit valid research using coded data.

ICD-9-CM and Its Current Application

Starting with the seventh edition of ICD, adaptations or modifications have been made in the United States for use in health care facilities. The ICD-9-CM is currently used by health care facilities for coding and reimbursement and by the state and federal agencies that are responsible for preparing vital statistics on births, deaths, and fetal deaths. Long-term care facilities may also report ICD-9-CM codes for reimbursement on Medicare and other federal patients.

ICD-9-CM is a statistical classification system designed to furnish quantitative diagnostic and procedural data on groups of cases. However, it does not contain nomenclature that allows for specific descriptions of all approved clinical and pathological terminology. HIM professionals must work with the variety of diagnostic and procedural terminologies that are used within a health care facility. These may be traced to the terminology patterns of various medical schools or clinical specialties related to the physicians on the staff and to their age group.

ICD-9-CM accommodates all terms—standard or colloquial, old or new—in classifying information from vital records and inpatient and outpatient health records.

ICD-9-CM represents a series of necessary compromises among classifications based on etiology, anatomical site, age, and circumstances of onset. It was developed to provide a statistical compilation of illnesses and injuries. In addition, it provides a supplemental classification for factors influencing health status and contact with health services (the V codes), a supplemental classification for external causes of injuries (the E codes), and a classification of surgical and nonsurgical procedures (the procedure index).

Diseases are grouped according to the problems they present, with specific disease entities given separate titles or code numbers only when their separation is warranted. Frequency of occurrence or importance as a morbid condition justifies assigning a separate category. Conditions of lesser frequency or importance are grouped together, often as residual groups of diseases of a particular anatomical site or physiological system. This arrangement results in a relatively simple numerical code and a statistical classification that serves the most important needs of the health care institution.

The CMS requires that health care facilities use ICD-9-CM in reporting diagnostic and procedural data as a prerequisite for payment of services provided to Medicare recipients. The ICD-9-CM codes serve as the basis for DRGs, which are the foundation of PPSs implemented by Medicare and some Medicaid programs. The ICD-9-CM code(s) determines the DRG into which the patient falls, and payment is based on the DRG. State Medicaid agencies also require health care facilities to use ICD-9-CM in reporting data for reimbursement purposes, as do most third-party payers.

Ambulatory care providers, including clinics, surgery centers, and physicians' offices, are required to use ICD-9-CM to report diagnoses on claim forms for Medicare patients and others. The *Medicare Carrier's Manual*, Section 4020.2, lists CMS coding and reporting requirements for physician billing and outlines the appropriate use of the ICD-9-CM system for physicians.[6]

Coding Resources and the Cooperating Parties

ICD-9-CM contains three sections: a tabular list, an alphabetical index, and the procedure classification. Various editions can be ordered from many publishers, including the U.S. Government Printing Office.

The American Hospital Association maintains a central office regarding the ICD-9-CM, in cooperation with the U.S. Public Health Service's National Center for Health Statistics and AHIMA, to answer coding questions and to promote the correct use of ICD-9-CM among health care facilities. The AHA publishes educational materials for use by health care facilities and educational institutions in training personnel to code with ICD-9-CM. The AHA's publications include the *ICD-9-CM Coding Handbook*[7] and the *Coding Clinic for ICD-9-CM*—a quarterly technical newsletter that contains current information on coding.[8] New in 2001, the AHA is offering *Coding Clinic for HCPCS*—a quarterly newsletter for HCPCS level-I and level-II facility reporting. All of the coding information in the *Coding Clinic* is published with the written approval of all of the cooperating parties: the AHA, AHIMA, CMS, and the National Center for Health Statistics.

The ICD-9-CM Coordination and Maintenance Committee is a federal interdepartmental committee charged with maintaining and updating the ICD-9-CM system. Suggestions for code modifications can come from the public and private sectors or from individuals or organizations. A cross-walk is being developed by CMS to assist in moving from ICD-9-CM to the new ICD-10-CM.

ICD-9-CM and DRGs in Reimbursement

Virtually all HIM departments use a computerized system, or grouper program, to classify patients into appropriate DRGs. Encoding systems, or computerized coding systems, are also used by many institutions, and programs are available from a variety of vendors. Various software options include coding, grouping, editing, and optimizing. Branching logic is typically used to lead the coder to the most accurate, specific code. Software programs can yield greater coding consistency from the coding staff and are updated regularly as coding changes occur. Programs are also available to simultaneously code both the ICD-9-CM code required for inpatients with the CPT codes required in the outpatient setting. A program for DRG management can be separate or integrated with an encoding system. Using a computerized program with multiple groupers, extensive editing, and optimizers can significantly improve reimbursement.

Originally, the DRG system was not designed as a payment system but rather as a managerial system. The use of DRGs in areas other than reimbursement includes physician profiling and the identification of areas for quality improvement and management planning. The coding and classification functions of the HIM department have become more complex because of the implementation of PPS-based DRGs. The basic DRG concept remains one in which patients can be categorized into groups on the basis of various factors, such as their diagnoses and treatment, age, and their statistically similar lengths of stay. The HIM professional must be knowledgeable in the various case-mix classification systems used to measure the categories of patients and the types of patients treated by a health care institution.

DRGs and Their Application for Severity

A criticism of DRGs has been that the system does not take into account the severity of a patient's disease. Severity-of-illness methodologies go beyond DRGs in order to classify to what degree a patient is sick. Clinical differences in patients with the same diagnosis can account for varying levels of care being rendered and varying amounts of resources being used. HIM professionals must be aware of current severity-of-illness systems available for health care facility use. The systems available use a combination of the principal diagnosis and various other factors (including secondary diagnoses, surgical procedures, age, sex, and clinical course) to determine a patient's severity or acuity level. Once a severity system is adopted by an institution, then data such as costs can be compared within DRGs in relation to severity. Valuable clinical and financial data are available for specific patient groupings. The HIM professional is a key player in these data management activities.

Payers are increasingly using severity-adjusted data to compare health care facilities. This type of comparison requires correct data. Insufficient coding detail and specificity could, for example, have a negative impact on a managed care contract, showing less acuity than actually exists at the facility.

ICD-9-CM and Outpatient Reimbursement

Ambulatory care providers, including clinics and physicians' offices, are required to use ICD-9-CM to report diagnoses on claim forms for Medicare patients and for patients insured by other carriers. Payment is no longer determined solely by the procedure code but rather by linking the correct ICD-9-CM code to the correct procedure code. This linkage communicates to the carrier the exact procedure or service (CPT-HCPCS code) performed and the reason (ICD-9-CM code). Medicare and other carriers now closely scrutinize claims to ensure that the ICD-9-CM code provided for a service supports the need or reflects the "medical necessity" for the service. For a claim to be paid by a carrier, each procedure must be linked to a medically necessary diagnosis. If in doubt of an appropriate linkage, the coder should seek clarification from the clinician. Medicare publishes "Local Medical Review Policies" (LMRPs) in their bulletins and on their Web site. LMRPs detail coverage limitations and diagnoses for many procedures and services. Coders should be familiar with LMRPs and educate clinical staff on Medicare requirements for specified services.

Oncology

The *International Classification of Diseases—Oncology* (ICD-O) is a publication of the WHO that provides for coding of the extensive topography, morphology (histology), and behavior of tumors.[9] Although ICD-9-CM contains a principally topographic code for neoplasms, with an arrangement to identify the tumor's behavior (malignant, benign, in situ, and so forth), it identifies only a few tumors by histological type.

ICD-O is divided into three sections. The first contains codes ranging from 140.0 to 199.9 that are used to identify sites in the body where a tumor might be located. The second—a "Morphology–Numerical List"—contains codes that are used to specify the type of tumor and its behavior. (The first four numbers of this code specify the histology, and the fifth number, following the slash, specifies the behavior.) The third section contains an alphabetical index to assess these neoplasm codes. ICD-O is used in cancer registry programs and other programs that require additional specificity in the tumor code.

Mental Disorders

The *Diagnostic and Statistical Manual of Mental Disorders*, 4th Edition (DSM-IV-TR), is a statistical classification and glossary of mental disorders. The primary purpose of the American Psychiatric Association publication is to provide clear descriptions of diagnostic categories in order for clinicians to diagnose, study, and treat various mental disorders.[10]

The DSM-IV-TR system features diagnostic criteria, a multiaxial approach to the evaluation of mental disorders, expanded descriptions of disorders, and additional categories not included in ICD-9. (It also eliminates some categories contained in ICD-9.) DSM-IV-TR categories are more specific than ICD-9 codes and are designed to reflect the most current knowledge regarding mental disorders. It is not completely compatible with ICD-9, although the original intent of the DSM task force was to maintain compatibility.

DSM-IV-TR is used in psychiatric institutions and psychiatric units of health care facilities for indexing records by mental disorder and for compiling statistical data on patient care. Because ICD-9-CM must be used in Medicare and Medicaid reimbursement reporting, HIM professionals working in psychiatric institutions and health care facilities with psychiatric units need a working knowledge of both ICD-9-CM and DSM-IV-TR.

Other Nomenclatures and Classification Systems

The *Systematized Nomenclature of Medicine Reference Terminology* (SNOMED RT) is a publication of the American College of Pathologists.[11] It contains the most comprehensive nomenclature currently available. SNOMED RT is designed for computer storage and for the automatic encoding of medical text. The system is used by some anatomical pathology laboratories, as well as laboratory information system vendors and several managed care corporations. Many computer-based patient record system experts believe that SNOMED RT is particularly well suited for use in CPR systems. The system incorporates the ICD-9-CM terms and codes, and it is possible to cross-walk from SNOMED RT to ICD-9-CM.

The *Index for Radiologic Diagnoses* is a publication of the American College of Radiology.[12] It contains a classification system for diagnostic radiology departments. The code number describes both the anatomical site of the X-ray and the pathology of the disease. The amount of detail used in the code is left to the discretion of the facility.

Common Procedure Coding System
for Health Care Facilities and Ambulatory Care

Since 1987, health care facilities have been required to use HCFA's Common Procedure Coding System (HCPCS), including CPT, for reporting outpatient surgical services provided to Medicare beneficiaries. Physicians' offices and ambulatory care facilities have been using the CPT coding system since 1966. The HCPCS consists of two levels: (1) current procedural terminology and (2) national codes.

Level One: Current Procedural Terminology (CPT). Physicians' *Current Procedural Terminology* is a publication of the American Medical Association that lists nearly eight thousand medical and surgical procedures and services performed by physicians. It is updated and published annually by the AMA.[13] Codes from the surgery section of CPT are used for outpatient surgery reporting by health care facilities, and the entire system is used in ambulatory care.

Current Procedural Terminology was originally used to report medical services and procedures performed by physicians. Today, the purpose of CPT is to provide uniform terminology for accurately designating medical, surgical, and diagnostic services for use in communications among physicians, patients, and third parties. As such, CPT is used in payment systems for services provided by physicians. Each service and procedure is identified with a five-digit code.

The main body of the book is arranged in six sections, with corresponding subsections and subheadings. The sections cover the following areas:

- Evaluation and management
- Anesthesiology
- Surgery
- Radiology (including nuclear medicine and diagnostic ultrasound)
- Pathology and laboratory
- Medicine (except anesthesiology)

The physician using CPT terminology and coding selects the name of the procedure or service that most accurately identifies the service performed. Using CPT, the physician can report, in coded form, the place and type of physician-patient encounter, the diagnostic procedure performed, and the surgical procedures performed. The health record must reflect the service or procedure that is billed by the physician.

CMS has established CPT as the national standard code set for physician services. To improve the structure and process of CPT and to address the needs of the user community, CPT is undergoing significant changes. The fourth edition of CPT is currently in use in the United States. In advance of the significant changes expected in the fifth edition, the AMA is introducing two new categories of CPT codes: Category II codes for tracking performance measurements and Category III codes for tracking new and emerging technologies.[14] The traditional CPT codes are now considered Category I.

Use of Category II codes is optional and not required for correct coding or reimbursement. By coding elements of performance measures, information by which carriers assess quality patient care can be supplied more efficiently through administrative reports rather than time-consuming chart reviews or site surveys. Category II codes are planned for inclusion in CPT 2003 and will be located in a separate section of CPT following the Medicine section of Category I codes.

Category III codes are temporary codes used for tracking new and emerging technologies. The purpose of these codes is to facilitate data collection on new services to substantiate widespread use, clinical efficacy or in the FDA approval process. Reimbursement is based on carrier policy and not on an established yearly fee schedule as with Category I codes. Category III codes made their debut in CPT 2002 and, like Category II codes, they are located in a separate section of CPT, following the Medicine section of Category I codes.

Level Two: National Codes (Alphanumeric HCFA Codes). Medicare created national codes for use by physicians, non-physician health care practitioners, and supply vendors to supplement CPT in reporting services and supplies provided to Medicare recipients. The codes are updated annually by CMS. They are alphanumeric codes that begin with a letter, A through V, followed by four numbers. Physicians' offices are now required

Health Information Management

to use these codes for supplemental services when filing claims for reimbursement to Medicare and commercial carriers. For example, carriers prefer the more specific HCPCS Level II code rather than the general CPT code 99070 to reimburse for supplies.

Some Medicare intermediaries have developed local codes for use in particular regions. However, HIPAA's Final Rule supports eliminating the local codes and using a national standard code set. The CPT Category III codes will likely replace the local codes.[15]

Health care facilities use CPT codes to report all outpatient procedures except for out-of-scope and noncovered procedures (such as venipuncture, catheter insertion, and cosmetic surgery). With the exception of these procedures, health care facilities are required to report CPT codes for all other surgical procedures performed on outpatients, including those approved for ambulatory surgical centers (ASCs) and other significant surgical procedures that are not approved for ASCs.

HIM professionals need expertise in the CPT and HCPCS coding systems for internal health care facilities, physicians' offices, group practices, and managed care centers so that they may serve as resource persons to the medical staff. Coders need skills in coding, assessing the quality of coded data, and developing reports based on those data. In addition, the HIM professional needs excellent skills in data retrieval, analysis, and presentation. Managed care plans must demonstrate that their contracted providers are delivering high-quality care at a low cost. Complete and accurate coding of all health care data is more crucial than ever before.

Coding software packages for clinics and physician offices can greatly improve coding accuracy and compliance with coding guidelines. Software can verify that the ICD-9, HCPCS, and CPT codes are valid, that modifiers are used appropriately, and that the ICD-9-CM code is linked to the correct CPT-HCPCS code. These systems, when managed by knowledgeable HIM professionals, can assist with compliance activities by identifying problems before a claim is generated to the carrier. This allows the organization an opportunity to proactively resolve the problem and submit a correct claim for payment, thereby improving reimbursement and compliance.

RESOURCE-BASED RELATIVE VALUE SCALE

The Resource-Based Relative Value Scale, implemented on January 1, 1992, is the method of payment for physicians' services under Medicare Part B. The RBRVS is based on a national fee schedule and replaces the method previously used by Medicare since 1965. The previous system was called the "customary, prevailing, and reasonable charge" payment method. In contrast, the RBRVS system bases fees on the relative amounts of physician resources that are used to provide services. The CMS used a phase-in approach over the past three years to convert from the historical charge system to the resource-based RBRVS; 2002 marks the first year of a fully implemented resource-based reimbursement schedule.

Relative values have been established for CPT codes, and factors such as the work involved, the practice expense, and the malpractice insurance premiums are figured into the price that the physician receives for performing a procedure on a Medicare patient. The system recognizes that the cost of practicing medicine varies by geographical region. Adjustments are made to the relative value units as a result of changes in medical practice, coding changes, new data on relative value components, or the addition of new procedures. Additions and revisions to the relative value units are officially announced through publication of a final notice each year in the *Federal Register.*

Significant changes were made in the CPT coding system to coincide with RBRVS changes in reimbursement. This change in payment methodology marked a significant adjustment for all physicians, regardless of their clinical specialties. Many third party payers' payments to physicians are based on a negotiated fee schedule using payer-adjusted RVUs for CPT codes. Because of this, the HIM professional working in either acute or ambulatory care needs expertise in coding, billing, and reimbursement methodologies for Medicare and third-party payers. With this knowledge, HIM professionals are a vital asset to the health care organization's managed care contracting team.

Coding Quality

The quality of coded data is an issue of major importance to the HIM professional, the health care facility, and the HIM profession. Correct coding is crucial in data management, reimbursement, and other related issues. The 1996 AHIMA board of directors approved a position statement, "Quality Healthcare Data and Information" endorsing the concept of a need for accurate, consistently coded data. In an effort to improve the accuracy of the coding and DRG assignments performed at a health care facility, many HIM departments utilize prebilling or concurrent DRG reviews. For example, the DRG analyst or prebiller may be an employee of the department or work for an outside contracted service. This individual reviews the codes and DRGs selected by the department coders prior to billing. In addition, educational sessions are held with the coders on a regular basis (perhaps daily) to review the findings of the prebiller and to improve the decision making for the coders in the future. Weekly or monthly reports are generated to provide information on dollars gained or lost in the review process. The bottom line for the department is that effective quality control systems result in effective collection and management of clinical data to support optimal DRG-based reimbursement. The concurrent review process allows mistakes to be caught before a claim is filed. Education of the physician or the coder can then take place immediately.

Coders in physician offices should review superbills or charge tickets for accuracy and provide in-service training to the clinical staff on documentation, as well as changes in codes and coding requirements. Coders can also conduct prospective audits to review physician documentation against the evaluation and management code selected by the doctor for the office visit or consultation. The amount of documentation in the history, the physical examination, and the medical decision making must support the CPT evaluation and management code that is selected. The credentialed coder or HIM professional can provide guidance in this area, which also serves to improve organization compliance with health care laws.

Accurately coded data give providers the ability to measure clinical and financial results while supplying payers and managed care companies with the information they need to make payment and perform outcome analysis. Thus accurate information about health care practices and utilization is crucial to the success of the health care facility and to those involved in paying the claims. CMS's Partnerships for Quality Services Demonstration Project (formerly the Centers of Excellence Demonstration) illustrates the importance of complete and accurate health care data in a non-DRG environment. Under this program, special Medicare status is given to facilities that meet high volume and quality standards for selected services.[16] Reimbursement is then made in a single, bundled payment covering all inpatient health care facility and physician services. This also replaces DRG reimbursement. The end result produces increased volume that leads to improved quality of care and reduced health care costs. The program is currently limited to certain cardiovascular and orthopedic procedures.

Many activities, then, that are essential to a health care organization's success depend on the accuracy and integrity of the coded health care data, including—but not limited to—the following issues:[17]

- Strategic planning
- Quality of care
- Outcomes analysis
- Reimbursement
- Critical pathway development
- Wellness initiatives
- Utilization monitoring
- Statistical and financial analysis
- Research
- Case management and case-mix analysis
- Marketing and allocation of resources

- Economic credentialing

- Identification of "best practices"

- Practice pattern analysis

- Performance comparisons with other health care organizations

- Clinical decision support

Coding Ethics and Optimization in Coding

The linkage of coding systems to the reimbursement system has created ethical issues for the HIM professional. "Upcoding," or selecting a more intensive code than was actually performed or that exaggerates the patient's actual condition, must be avoided. AHIMA has developed the Standards of Ethical Coding to guide coders in the coding process. The coder is expected to strive for the optimal payment to which the facility is legally entitled, but it is considered unethical and illegal to maximize payment by means that contradict regulatory guidelines.

When coding for reimbursement, the employee must understand that the codes are the communication device between the facility and the third-party payer. Correctly coded data are crucial to the inpatient and outpatient aspects of a health care enterprise. Physicians should be consulted for clarification if they enter conflicting or ambiguous documentation in the chart, and the information therein must be adequate and appropriate to support the diagnoses and procedure codes selected.

AHIMA has issued a position statement regarding the association's role in prospective payment. It states, in part, that "inevitably, occasions arise when two qualified coders make different judgments in diagnosis classification and code assignments."[18] Recognizing that this can occur, employees must be committed to coding data according to the accepted conventions of the coding system they are using. There will be variables, such as the type and amount of documentation in the health record and in an individual's interpretation of the guidelines. The AHIMA Code of Ethics also speaks to the integrity of the HIM professional by stating in Code II that "Health information management professionals comply with all laws, regulations, and standards governing the practice of health information management."[19] Regardless of any pressure from a superior, the HIM professional must refuse to intentionally "upcode," or code to any inappropriate DRG for the sake of payment. Coding guidelines published by the CMS must be followed at all times.

Optimization involves selecting the most resource-intensive codes for a particular encounter while still following all the rules. Coders may legitimately optimize reimbursement by performing a complete review of the health record to identify all diagnoses and procedures to which physician or facility services can be coded and documented. Maximization, however, involves manipulating the sequence of codes or adding other codes (for comorbid conditions that are not substantiated in the record) in order to receive higher reimbursement. The HIM professional must refuse to maximize coding and instead abide by coding guidelines that support ethical practices.

Compliance in Coding

Adhering to the AHIMA Code of Ethics and insisting on high-quality coded data helps to obtain correct reimbursement for services and reduces the risks to the health care facility of committing health care fraud. There are a number of laws that protect health care benefit programs from fraud and abuse. Most laws apply to both federal and other third-party-payer programs.

CMS defines *fraud* as "an intentional deception or misrepresentation that someone makes, knowing it is false, that could result in an unauthorized payment." The attempt itself is fraudulent, whether or not it was successful.

Abuse is defined as "actions that are inconsistent with accepted, sound medical, business or fiscal practices." This practice also results in an unnecessary cost to the Medicare program.[20]

A health care facility can suffer severe financial consequences as a result of committing health care fraud. In addition to refunding all overpayments, penalties for violating Health Care Fraud laws can include substantial fines, exclusion from the Medicare program and, depending on the severity of the violation, prison terms for the perpetrators of the fraudulent scheme. The Office of Inspector General (OIG), under the direction of the U.S. Department of Health and Human Services (DHHS), investigates and prosecutes cases of suspected health care fraud. All health care facilities must take appropriate steps to ensure compliance with health care laws and regulations. The OIG recommends that each health care facility develop and implement a voluntary compliance program to identify and correct any potentially fraudulent or abusive practices in an organization. The OIG publishes compliance program guidance in the *Federal Register* and currently has published guidance for hospitals, clinical laboratories, home health agencies, durable medical equipment suppliers, individual and small group physician practices, third-party medical billing companies, hospices, nursing facilities, and Medicare+Choice organizations offering coordinated care plans.[21] It is beneficial to begin with the OIG's recommended compliance plan components as a base and then tailor a program to fit the needs of the organization.

The following are an example of OIG-recommended components for an effective compliance plan. Similar components are included in all of the compliance program guidances.[22]

- Conducting internal monitoring and auditing
- Implementing compliance and practice standards
- Designating a compliance officer or contact
- Conducting appropriate training and education
- Responding appropriately to detected offenses and developing corrective action
- Developing open lines of communication
- Enforcing disciplinary standards through well-publicized guidelines

It is vital that health care organizations understand the significance of health care fraud laws and the importance of balancing correct reimbursement with compliance with those laws. Employers must be sure that appropriately credentialed, trained, and qualified individuals perform coding and compliance functions. HIM professionals have a thorough understanding of coding, documentation, and reimbursement rules and are uniquely positioned to play a key role in developing, implementing, and managing a health care organization's compliance plan.

Coder Credentialing

The government's focus on health care fraud and abuse has created a significant need in the marketplace for credentialed coders who can improve the quality and accuracy of coding. AHIMA administers two such credentialing exams, one for coders based in health care facilities and one for those based in physician offices. (The rules and guidelines for each type of coder are different enough to warrant separate coding certification examinations.) Each exam, in addition to requiring actual coding, tests for the knowledge and understanding of data integrity, coding guidelines, coding quality, as well as the regulatory guidelines of the CMS and the policies of other payers. The credentials reflected in CCS and CCS-P status signify that the individual has successfully completed these examinations and has demonstrated mastery-level coding knowledge. Individuals already credentialed by AHIMA as RHITs or RHIAs are also eligible to take the coding specialist exams. Upon successful completion of these exams, the RHIT or RHIA may then use both designations.

A new entry-level coding credential—the CCA (certified coding associate)—has been approved for coders who are new to the field and lack the years of experience and knowledge required of the higher-level CCS and CCS-P credential. This credential will help employers identify those professionals with the appropriate level of knowledge and skill base to meet their needs. To sit for the entry-level coding certification exam, candidates are required to have a diploma from a U.S. high school. It is also recommended that the candidate have at least six months' experience in hospital inpatient and ambulatory care coding or successfully pass an AHIMA-approved coding certification program.[23]

Current Issues in Working with Coding and Classification Systems

With the advent of changes in health care delivery have come new HIM issues. Among those currently affecting the work of HIM professionals are case-mix management, managed care, and ambulatory patient classifications, and technological advancements.

Case-Mix Management. The DRG system for health care facilities and the RBRVS system for the physician's office created a new awareness regarding the importance of case-mix management. The categories of patients (including both type and volume) that are treated by a facility—the case-mix—represent the complexity of the facility's total caseload. As health information systems have become more sophisticated and clinical data have been merged with financial data, case-mix analysis has come to the forefront as a management tool.

Reports that are generated in case-mix management can be very simple or very complex. Data are generated to show the number of patients in a DRG and reimbursement per DRG. Data specific to charges within a DRG can also be computed, and these data can be related to a physician's practice. Accurate assessments of the vast amount of data generated require data interpretation skills. The HIM professional is responsible for ensuring that clinical and case-mix data that are generated from the HIM department are used appropriately and effectively by the health care institution's administration and medical staff

Managed Care. Managed care at the national level strives to control costs while increasing access to care. Managed competition today means partnerships among doctors, health care facilities, and insurers to provide health care to consumers in a cost-effective manner. The Group Health Association of America defines managed care as "that body of organizational, financial, and management activities that should be implemented by professionals and any organizational entity that is at financial risk for the cost of medical or surgical services they provide."[24] It is based on the principle of providing comprehensive primary care with reduced costs.

HIM professionals are familiar with health maintenance organizations (HMOs) as an example of managed care. The ambulatory care arena now demands the expertise of the HIM professional in interpreting coding issues relative to the various contracts of managed care plans (HMOs, PPOs, and others) operating within the health care institution. Managers must be responsive when managed care providers or the federal government request health information systems data for use in administering and evaluating programs that manage care. The HIM professional must also be proactive and assist his or her health care facility in evaluating the value of these contracts both operationally and financially to ensure written agreement with coding conventions and standard reimbursement methodologies.

Ambulatory Patient Classifications

Ambulatory patient classifications (APCs) were developed by 3M Health Information Systems under a contract with CMS. CMS identified APCs as the basis of a new outpatient prospective payment system for Medicare beneficiaries. Ambulatory patient classifications constitute an ambulatory case-mix system used for prospective payment in ambulatory care. The system is a patient-classification scheme designed to explain the amount and types of resources used in an ambulatory visit. Patients in each APC have similar clinical characteristics, resource use, and costs, and the APC describes the complete range of services provided in the outpatient setting. The APC system packages a facility's payment for outpatient services, and therefore providers may experience decreased reimbursement for the same services as compared with existing outpatient payment methodologies. APCs require providers to review coding practices to ascertain that they are receiving adequate reimbursement to cover costs. APCs were officially implemented nationwide in August 2001.

Multiple APCs can be assigned to an outpatient during a single visit.[25] The ICD-9-CM diagnosis codes drive the assignment of a medical APC, whereas the CPT-HCPCS procedure code drives the procedural and ancillary APCs. APC software is currently available from 3M Health Information Systems to help ambulatory care organizations determine outpatient payment and verify payment received, as well as to evaluate costs and resource use.

TECHNOLOGY ADVANCEMENTS IN CODING

Technological advances are bringing the heath care industry into the digital age. Capabilities of current computerized coding applications have geographical and functional implications for the coding professional. Web-based solutions are now used by many facilities to support home-based coders and to outsource coding functions. Electronic medical record (EMR) technology facilitates coding closer to the point of service by digitizing clinical data so that CPT and ICD-9 codes can be assigned directly from physician orders and dictation. Coders can then verify the accuracy of the codes assigned by the system. Claim scrubber software programs are available that analyze claims for correct CPT and ICD-9 coding. Coders provide database management support for these programs by using their knowledge to tailor the system to their organization and local payer requirements. HIM professionals are skilled in analyzing health care data and can use the information collected through the claim scrubber software to prioritize coding training needs and establish objective performance measures. Auto-coding technology is being developed that extracts diagnosis and procedure codes directly from dictated reports. This technology shows promise for specialties with homogenous data forms such as radiology reports.[26] Coding performed by automated systems must be reviewed by knowledgeable coding professionals to assure accuracy and compliance with coding guidelines.

Technology is streamlining the technical aspect of coding and creating new opportunities for coders and the HIM profession. There is a greater need for high-level coders in oversight and quality assurance roles to verify that the automated systems are assigning codes accurately and optimizing reimbursement in compliance with health care regulations. HIM professionals must continuously learn about technological advancements that can improve coding accuracy and efficiency. By proactively bringing technology into their organization, HIM professionals assume a leadership role in the organization's management team.

CONCLUSION

It has been many years since the advent of the PPS and DRGs. The HIM professional has faced significant challenges during this period and will continue to do so in the future. The quality of clinical data submitted by all health care institutions is crucial to the future of the health care delivery system. The accuracy of clinical data abstracting and coding significantly affects health care facilities.

Coding will continue to change in the computer-based patient record environment, and new systems will most likely be put in place. Furthermore, the profession may be more involved in managing the computerized coding and encoding systems than in assigning codes directly.

The key to survival in the world of decreasing reimbursement and increased regulations will be the successful partnership of health information managers with enlightened health care providers and facility administrators who embrace the philosophy of consistent, high-quality data.

REFERENCES

1. *Health Care Financing Administration, International Classification of Diseases, 9th Revision, Clinical Modification* (Washington, D.C.: Department of Health and Human Services, Public Health Service, HCFA, 2001).
2. American Medical Association, *Physicians' Current Procedural Terminology* 2001 Edition (Chicago: AMA, 2001).
3. Centers for Medicare and Medicaid Services, "ICD-9-CM Coding for Diagnostic Tests," Program Memorandum, Change Request 1724, Transmittal AB-01-144 (Baltimore, Md.: CMS, September 26, 2001).
4. D. Pickett, *Society for Clinical Coding 2000 Annual Meeting Presentation Highlights* (Chicago: September 23–24, 2000). On-line; available at www.sccoding.org/codewrite/Jan-feb01
5. R. Averill, R. Mullin, B. Steinbeck, N. Goldfield, and T. Grant (May 1998), "Development of the ICD-10 Procedure Coding System (ICD-10-PCS)."

Journal of AHIMA, May 1998. On-line; available at www.ahima.org/journal/coding/coding.9805.html

6. Centers for Medicare and Medicaid Services, "Claims Review and Adjudication Procedures," *Medicare Carriers Manual*, Part 3, Section 4020 (2): 4–20, 4.

7. Faye Brown, in cooperation with the Central Office on ICD-9-CM of the American Hospital Association, *ICD-9-CM Coding Handbook*, 1997 Rev. Ed. (Chicago: American Hospital Publishing, Inc., 1997). (Available with or without answers.)

8. American Hospital Association, *Coding Clinic for ICD-9-CM* (Chicago: American Hospital Association). Published quarterly.

9. World Health Organization, *International Classification of Diseases for Oncology*, 2nd ed. (Geneva, Switzerland: WHO, 1990).

10. American Psychiatric Association, *Diagnostic and Statistical Manual-IV-TR* (Washington, D.C.: APA, 2000).

11. College of American Pathologists, *Systematized Nomenclature of Medicine International Reference Terminology* (Northfield, Ill.: CAP, 2000).

12. American College of Radiology, *Index for Radiology Diagnoses*, 4th ed. (Chicago: ACR, 1999).

13. American Medical Association, *Physicians' Current Procedural Terminology 2001 Edition* (Chicago: AMA, 2001).

14. American Medical Association, *Current Procedural Terminology (CPT) Category II and Category III Codes Informational Report*. Proceedings of the Interim 2000 Meeting of the AMA House of Delegates, Report of the Board of Trustees, 36-I-00. (Orlando, Fl.: December 2000).

15. Ibid.

16. S. Prophet and G. Bryant, "Growing Demand for Accurate Coded Data in New Healthcare Delivery Era," *Journal of AHIMA* 68, no. 1 (January 1997): 42.

17. Ibid.

18. American Medical Record Association, *Coding Competency: A Position Statement of the American Medical Record Association* (Chicago: AMRA, 1984).

19. AHIMA, "American Health Information Management Association Code of Ethics," Amended December 1991, *Journal of AHIMA* 63, no. 1 (January 1992): 94.

20. Federal Register, "OIG Compliance Program for Individual and Small Group Physician Practices," 65, no. 194 (October 5, 2000): 59434–59452.

21. Ibid.

22. Ibid.

23. "House of Delegates 2001: Coding at the Crossroads." *AHIMA Advantage*, 5, no. 5 (October 2001): 5.

24. C. Boester, "What Is This Thing Called Managed Care?" *Journal of AHIMA* 64, no. 7 (July 1993): 61.

25. Richard F. Averill, Thelma M. Grant, and Barbara A. Steinbeck, "Preparing for the Outpatient Prospective Payment System," *Journal of AHIMA* (July/August 2000). On-line; available at www.ahima.org/journal/features/feature.0007.2.html

26. M. Hagland, "Revolution in Progress: How Technology is Reshaping the Coding World." *Journal of AHIMA* 73, no. 7 (July/August 2002): 32–35.

BIBLIOGRAPHY

Abdelhak, Mervat, ed. *Health Information: Management of a Strategic Resource.* Philadelphia: W.B. Saunders, 1996.

Chidley, E. "Medicare: The Correct Coding Initiative." *For the Record* 9, no. 5 (March 10, 1997): 7.

Dill, E. "Mastering the APG Grouping Process." *For the Record* 9, no. 7 (April 7, 1997): 12.

Duncan, D., and Goldfield, N. "Case-Mix Measurements for Understanding and Managing Healthcare Institutions." *Journal of AHIMA* 64, no. 7 (July 1993): 44.

Ferconio, S., and Yoder, L. "Managing the Business of Ambulatory Care: The Emerging Role of Health Information Managers." *Journal of AHIMA* 64, no. 7 (July 1993): 55.

Fox, L. "An Ethical Dilemma: Coding Medical Records for Reimbursement." *Journal of AHIMA* 63, no. 1 (January 1992): 34.

Huffman, E. *Health Information Management,* 10th ed. Berwyn, Ill.: Physicians' Record Company, 1994.

Prophet, S. "AHIMA Provides Testimony on Coding/Classification Issues Pertaining to HIPAA Implementation." *Journal of AHIMA* 68, no. 7 (July/August 1997): 52.

_____. "Classification Systems: Taking a Broader Look." *Journal of AHIMA* 68, no. 5 (May 1997): 46.

Whalen, L., and Jones, D. "Pre-Billing DRG Reviews Set New Standard." *Journal of AHIMA* 64, no. 7 (July 1993): 58.

CHAPTER 9

Health Care Databases and Statistics

Nancy Coffman-Kadish

H ealth care institutions generate clinical and financial health care data to satisfy each facility's need for internal information and to meet the increasing requirements of data users outside the institutions. Data that are collected for a particular purpose are known collectively as a *database;* a database management system is used to store and retrieve the data. Efficient database management systems are essential for internal and external data needs.

Health care data maintained in a database management system are useful in a variety of applications. Patient care within an institution can best be evaluated and managed when adequate information is available regarding a large number of inpatients and ambulatory care patients and their treatment. Information about length-of-stay, diagnoses, therapies, tests, case outcomes, and procedures can be collected from individual records and analyzed to gauge the quality, effectiveness, and appropriate degree of care rendered by health care professionals.

At the national level, the incidence of specific illnesses and disabilities, life expectancies, and mortality rates are described by population-based statistics. Health care resources, including the supply of personnel, facilities, and services, can be described statistically. Resource statistics may be related to utilization statistics that pertain to inpatient services, ambulatory care, and the types of practices providing services. Information on health care costs, financing, and sources of expenditures is useful in an increasing variety of analyses.

Total quality management and continuous quality improvement techniques rely on the collection and management of meaningful statistical information in a database management system. Health care organizations are continuously requested to prove the quality of care that they provide, and statistically valid data are needed to support explanations regarding patterns of care and justifications for variations in care.

This chapter focuses on the major data sets that are used by health care institutions and provides a basic overview of major statistical terminology and techniques. In addition, the chapter examines the increasingly vital roles that HIM professionals have shouldered in meeting the needs of their health care organizations. Today's HIM professional may function as a clinical data specialist, a data quality manager, or a specialist in the research and decision support area. To successfully lead in these areas of practice, HIM professionals must have a well-developed knowledge of statistical measures, research study designs, and data analysis.

CLINICAL AND FINANCIAL HEALTH CARE DATA

Health care facilities base significant financial decisions on the data generated and maintained in the HIM department. The HIM professional plays an integral role in the implementation and use of the health care facility's information system because so much of the information originates in the patient record or is generated through related information that is managed by the HIM department. In addition to providing the data, the practitioner needs an awareness of data literacy, data integration, data quality, and the relationship of these data to financial variables such as case-mix, acuity, and severity of patient conditions.

The Financial-Clinical Database

The patient record is the crucial data source that enables the health care facility to address the issues of cost, quality, and patient outcomes. Clinical and financial database issues are complex because there may be multiple records for patients generated at multiple care sites, inconsistencies in format and data entry, no standard basis on which to compare protocols or results of procedures, and no data on ultimate outcomes. Clinical information, as documented in the patient record, is a key component of a health care facility's case-mix database under any prospective payment reimbursement system. The accuracy of the clinical and financial data affects a facility's management decisions and the viability of the organization.

Clinical Data Management

The role of the HIM department has changed dramatically since implementation of the Medicare prospective payment system (PPS) for inpatients in 1983 and for outpatients in 2000. Historically, health care facilities were paid on the basis of the patient's length of stay and the services rendered—information that was easily obtainable from various sources within the institution. Since the establishment of the PPS, however, payment has been calculated according to DRGs for inpatients and APCs for outpatients, which in turn is based on the documentation and coding in the health record. Under PPS, a primary function of the HIM professional is clinical data management, that is, ensuring that complete, timely, and accurate data are available for DRG and APC assignment and billing purposes. Late records, incorrect coding of diagnoses or procedures, or misinterpretation of the record content can lead to underpayment or overpayment for a patient's stay. Thus the role of the HIM department is crucial to the health care facility's financial operation. The size, skills, and performance levels of the department staff must be assessed with the requirements of Medicare PPS in mind.

The Joint Commission's *Comprehensive Accreditation Manual for Hospitals* states the following:

Uniform data definitions and data capture methods are used whenever possible. Minimum data sets . . . are standardized whenever possible. The hospital collects data in a timely, economic, and efficient manner and with the degree of accuracy, completeness, and discrimination necessary for their intended use. The hospital minimizes bias in the data and regularly assesses the data's reliability, validity, and accuracy.[1]

The HIM professional applies this statement to the information management process with the goal of converting data into information that is useful in the decision-making processes of the health care facility. In so doing, the practitioner must identify crucial information needs, define data elements, determine the data collection methodology, and collect the data. Additional steps, similar to those in a quality management program, include analyzing the data, displaying and presenting the data, interpreting and evaluating the information, and acting and reporting on the information. Finally, to manage clinical data effectively, the HIM professional needs to possess skills and knowledge in data integration, efficient data storage, and data security. Effective clinical data management skills allow for optimum communications between health care professionals and providers.

The information management focus of the Joint Commission regulations clearly charges the HIM professional with developing a management information system that meets internal and external information needs. The system's design should incorporate needs for data and information within and among departments, the medical staff, the administration, and the governing body, as well as information that is needed to support relationships with outside services, companies, and agencies.[2] Data need to be provided efficiently for patient care, education, and management. The additional challenge in the information system is the ability to link to external databases and to provide information for research purposes, as required by the facility. To accomplish this linkage, the HIM professional must be familiar with statistical techniques.

Health Information Management

Database Credibility and Integrity

The HIM professional is responsible for knowing where the needed data are located, how they are maintained, and who is maintaining them. An initial step in data integration is determining the clinical data set for the health care facility's information system, typically called a *data dictionary*. Definitions must be standardized for each data element of the database. To arrive at such definitions, health facilities can establish a team that includes the HIM department director, the chief financial officer, a representative from continuous quality improvement (CQI) or utilization management (UM), an administrator or a chief information officer, and a medical staff representative. This team would define the clinical data set that the health facility will maintain, determine the source or format of those data, and assume responsibility for designing a system to assess the quality of the data. With standards in place, the clinical information system of the facility becomes one that is accurate and appropriate.[3]

Data dictionaries that define the data elements are useful in standardizing the collected data. A complete dictionary describes such information as the field, the data's origin, applicable edits and rules, and security levels that apply to the field. Uniform data collection systems such as the Uniform Hospital Discharge Data Set (UHDDS) or the Uniform Ambulatory Care Data Set (UACDS), discussed in the following section, allow comparisons among the nation's health care facilities. These databases can be used by Quality Improvement Organizations (QIOs; formerly known as Peer Review Organizations, or PROs) to analyze each Medicare provider's pattern of care. Database management systems can provide in-depth clinical information for use in improving a facility's quality of care.

STANDARDIZED DATA SETS

Computerized database management systems make it possible for data from various sources to be linked for the purposes of analysis and comparison. To facilitate these comparisons, providers and users must follow a uniform system for reporting information. Uniform data sets that identify specific data elements that should be collected and descriptions that define their meanings exist for several health care settings.

Uniform Hospital Discharge Data Set

One of the first steps toward identifying, defining, and uniformly recording health care data took place in 1969, when the National Center for Health Statistics and The Johns Hopkins University sponsored a conference on hospital discharge abstract systems. The end result of this conference was the development and implementation of UHDDS, which serves as a minimum basic data set for reporting by all short-term general hospitals, that is, hospitals with patients who typically stay fewer than thirty days.

In 1974, the U.S. Department of Health, Education, and Welfare adopted UHDDS reporting as departmental policy for Medicare and Medicaid programs and their patient populations. The goal was to improve the uniformity and comparability of health care facility discharge data. Since that time, the system has undergone several revisions. To stay abreast of data requirements, HIM professionals should consult the latest editions of appropriate government publications, such as the *Federal Register* or state administrative codes. Currently, the data items to be included in the health records of all inpatients are listed as follows:

1. Patient identification (unique personal identification number—UPIN)
2. Date of birth (month, day, and year)
3. Sex
4. Race and ethnicity
5. Residence (full address and nine-digit ZIP code, if available)
6. Hospital identification number (the Medicare provider number is recommended)
7. Admission date (month, day, and year)
8. Type of admission (scheduled or unscheduled)

9. Discharge date (month, day, and year)

10. Attending physician identification—(UPIN)

11. Operating physician identification—(UPIN)

12. Principal diagnosis

13. Other diagnoses (all conditions that coexist at the time of admission or that develop subsequently that affect the treatment received or the length of stay)

14. Qualifier for other diagnoses (indicating whether the onset of the diagnosis preceded or followed admission to the health care facility)

15. External cause-of-injury code (if there has been a diagnosis of an injury, poisoning, or adverse effect)

16. Birth weight of neonate

17. Procedures and dates

18. Disposition of patient

19. Patient's expected source of payment

20. Total charges

Procedures are reported in accordance with the UHDDS definition of significant procedures and the ICD-9-CM procedure classification (see Chapter Eight). In addition, each physician should have a universally unique number across all health care facilities and data systems. The Medicare UPIN, which is recommended for this purpose, can be used to identify the attending and operating physicians. A permanent, unique number can be used by all providers and third-party payers for physicians and patients to link patients across care systems and permit creation of a longitudinal record.

The UHDDS items should be included in the records of all inpatients, but they do not constitute a complete health record. Some items are documented in records other than the individual patient health record—for example, the data on total charges. In such instances, a capability should exist to link data from the various data sources. This linkage is considered to be an essential aspect of the data set.

An advantage of the computer-based patient record is that it allows data from different sources to be linked. However, confidentiality is a concern. Programs and other organizations that collect and use such health data must assume responsibility for safeguarding it and protect citizens' rights under applicable laws and regulations. The Health Insurance Portability and Accountability Act (HIPAA) requires that health care facilities design and maintain systems to protect the security and privacy of electronically transmitted data. Such a system should prevent unauthorized individuals from accessing, creating, or modifying information while allowing authorized users to have access.

Ambulatory Care: Uniform Ambulatory Care Data Set

The National Committee on Vital and Health Statistics approved a minimum data set for ambulatory care records in 1989. The Uniform Ambulatory Care Data Set (UACDS) identifies essential data items that many federal health and funding programs require from providers as a condition of participation. The purpose of the data set is to improve the comparability of ambulatory care data by defining a common core of standard data items with uniform definitions. Data are collected in three major areas: (1) patient data items, (2) provider data items, and (3) encounter data items. Items that are maintained in the three areas of the data set include the following:

Patient Data Items
1. Personal identification
2. Residence
3. Date of birth (month, day, year)
4. Sex
5. Race and ethnic background
6. Living arrangement and marital status (optional)

Provider Data Items

1. Provider identification (name and UPIN)

2. Location or address

3. Profession (MD, DO, DDS, and so on)

Encounter Data Items

1. Date, place or site, and address of encounter (if different from item 8)

2. Patient's reason for encounter (optional)

3. Services (diagnostic, therapeutic, and preventive)

4. Disposition (no follow-up or follow-up planned)

5. Patient's expected sources of payment

6. Total charges

The increased focus on, and importance of, ambulatory care makes it essential for the HIM professional to establish systems for uniform collection and management of ambulatory care data.

Long-Term Care: Minimum Data Set and Resident Assessment Protocols

Because the length of stay in long-term care facilities can vary from a few months to several years, the amount of data collected is vast. The minimum data set (MDS) is under the control of the National Committee on Vital and Health Statistics (NCVHS) and assists long-term care facilities in their data collection efforts by ensuring that the data collected are uniform and comparable. The Minimum Data Set for Nursing Home Resident Assessment and Care Screening was originally developed in 1980 and updated in the late 1990s. The MDS is divided into sections that include not only identification and health items but items regarding the resident's background, cognitive abilities, behavioral patterns, and ability to perform the activities of daily living. This data set is rather lengthy and has not been listed. The HIM practitioner should consult the most recent version for the complete content and definitions.

Home Health: Outcome and Assessment Information Set

Home health services are becoming a vital link in the continuum of care. As the volume of home health visits increases, it is important to collect a standard set of data elements that can document the quality of care provided and verify services provided for reimbursement purposes. This data set was approved in regulations published in 1999 as a result of a mandate of the Omnibus Budget Reconciliation Act (OBRA) of 1987. This data set is also lengthy and divided into many sections, such as clinical record items, patient demographics and history, and living arrangements; several sections assess the patient's status of several body systems, such as integumentary and respiratory. The HIM practitioner should consult the most recent version for the complete content and definitions.

BASIC STATISTICAL TECHNIQUES

Statistical data can be used in research studies—for example, in identifying risk factors associated with the development of a disease or condition. Data can be calculated as a rate when there is a comparison of event frequency in one population with frequency of the same event in a comparable population. Some departments provide mortality and morbidity data in the form of rates. The latter might include the number or incidence of new cases of transfusion reactions of patients receiving blood during a certain year.

Descriptive Statistics

Health care facilities collect seemingly endless amounts of data. But after collecting all of the data, it is important to summarize and present them so they can be quickly understood and put to use. *Descriptive statistics* (a mean, median, or mode, for example) summarize data so that they describe the results of a particular study without making further inferences

184

about the results. The summary data can be displayed in graphs, tables, diagrams, and so on. The HIM practitioner must know the different types of data that may be collected and understand the meanings of various statistical terms in order to compile the data into a form that has meaning and can be used for decision making.

A *population* is a complete set of individuals, objects, or measurements that have a common characteristic. It is the group from which the sample, or subset, is selected. A sample should be selected in a random manner, meaning that each member of the population has an equal opportunity to be selected. Two other terms used are *constant* and *variable.*

A *constant* is a value that never changes; it is replaceable with one and only one value. A constant is one's date or place of birth, or it is the common factor that applies to everyone or everything in a population and sample. For example, in a study of patients who are discharged from the hospital with a diagnosis of emphysema, the constant is the diagnosis of emphysema.

A *variable* is a factor that assumes different values or outcomes. One variable can be studied, such as the age of the patients with emphysema. Or two or more variables can be compared, such as the age and smoking history of patients discharged with a diagnosis of emphysema.

Different kinds of data, which are either *categorical* or *numerical* in nature, are collected, summarized, and displayed in different ways. Categorical data have observations that can be characterized according to a characteristic or quality; they may be nominal or ordinal. Nominal data are values that fall into unordered categories. The sequence of the values is unimportant. Examples include variables such as sex, place of birth, and diagnostic category. Numbers may be used to represent categories; for example, "1" may represent male and "2" may represent "female." Ordinal data are types of data where either the sequence of the values is important or the order is ranked, such as the leading cause of death or the level of patient satisfaction.

Numerical data have numerical values and yield observations that can be expressed numerically, such as weight, blood pressure, number of deaths, and pulse rate. Numerical data can be further classified as either discrete or continuous. Discrete data are data with values that are finite, distinct, and separate, such as the number of deaths, admissions, or discharges. The numbers assume whole values because they represent individuals. Continuous data are data in an uninterrupted range of values, such as weight, blood pressure, and pulse rate, which has an upper and lower limit.

When summarizing the results of a study, it is often useful to indicate an "average" of the data collected from a population, or sample. Measures of central tendency—the mean, median, and mode—are used to locate the middle or typical value in a frequency distribution. The mean is the average; the median is the midpoint of all the values placed in rank order, and the mode is the value that occurs most frequently. The suitability of any one of the three measures depends on the situation under examination. The mean is the most common measure of central tendency because it can be used for further statistical analysis such as determining the variance and the standard deviation. A drawback of measuring the mean is that it can be skewed by very high or very low numbers. This can be compensated for by using the median to describe the average, as it is unaffected by extreme values. The choice of a measure of central tendency will depend on the number of values and the nature of the distribution. All three measures of central tendency may be used because they illustrate and describe data in different ways.

When a distribution of numbers is graphed, the shape of the lines or bars on the graph will also tell a lot about the distribution. A normal distribution, or "bell-shaped curve," means that the mean, median, and mode are identical and lie at the center of the distribution. If the majority of the values are grouped at either the low or high end of the values, the curve will be "skewed." A "tail" will form at the end in which the small number of values lie. The direction of the skewness refers to the location of the tail rather than the side in which the greater number of values are grouped. If the values are grouped at the high end of the distribution, the distribution is skewed to the left and is said to be negatively skewed. If the values are grouped at the low end of the distribution, the distribution is skewed to the right, or positively skewed.

In addition to measures of central tendency to describe a distribution of numbers, it is important to provide information about the amount of variability among the numbers. One such measure is the range—the difference between the highest and lowest values. Its major disadvantage is that it uses only two values from the data set and ignores all others.

Two other measures of data dispersion, in addition to the range, are the standard deviation and the variance. The standard deviation indicates how far the values are from the mean. The smaller the standard deviation, the smaller the variability, or the more the values cluster around the mean. The variance is very similar to the standard deviation in that it demonstrates how values are spread around the mean. The purpose of measuring variance is to compare the variability between two groups. However, comparisons may not be valid if the two groups have very different means.

The HIM professional might use several of the statistical techniques that are discussed in this section to perform a comparison study. For example, the length of stay for patients who have community-acquired pneumonia might be compared with that of patients who have nosocomial pneumonia (pneumonia acquired in the health care facility more than seventy-two hours after admission). Statistical techniques may also be used to uncover patterns or trends in a group of cases.

The HIM professional also needs expertise in data presentation techniques. The way that data are presented may determine whether an appropriate decision is made and appropriate action undertaken. Because clinical quality assessment and performance improvement are very dependent on the analysis of patterns and trends, the manner in which data are collected and displayed is crucial to the outcome and ultimate effectiveness of the process. Techniques such as chi-square distribution, t-test, and regression analysis can be used to compare groups of data.

A chi-square distribution compares two groups of raw data, or rates. It is used to determine whether an actual distribution differs from a predetermined, theoretical distribution. The results of a chi-square distribution identify the difference between comparable groups or conditions and the predicted rates of a particular occurrence or event. The *t*-test compares two means to determine whether they indicate real differences or a difference that is likely to have occurred by chance. Regression analysis allows the comparison of an entire distribution of observations or that of one variable with the entire distribution of another variable to determine the correlation between two variables. This type of analysis assumes the use of linear data, however, and its use may be limited.

Other terms are frequently used when referring to health statistics. The terms *incidence* and *prevalence* refer to diseases, or morbidity. *Incidence* indicates the number of new cases of a disease or condition that occur during a specified period of time. Incidence is typically used to describe acute conditions or diseases, such as measles. *Prevalence* is the number of existing cases of a disease, regardless of onset. Prevalence is typically used to describe chronic conditions, such as chronic obstructive pulmonary disease (COPD).

The concepts of *validity* and *reliability* are paramount to all statistical interpretation of data. *Validity* is the capability of a test or tool to measure what it is intended to measure. Correctly recorded ICD-9-CM diagnoses are an example of valid data. *Reliability* is the ability of a test or tool to measure in a reproducible way what it is intended to measure. The implication is that no matter how many times the data are collected, they will remain consistent. In coding and abstracting, each coder must follow the same guidelines for the coded data to be reliable.

Summarized data and a percentage of compliance or variation levels for a given set of criteria can be displayed for a particular department, diagnosis, procedure, and so on. Graphing techniques such as histograms, frequency polygons, bar graphs, pie charts, and Pareto charts can be used in data display. It is important to use the appropriate graph for the type of data to be presented. The type used depends on the type to be presented. Continuous numerical data should be presented on a histogram or frequency polygon, whereas categorical data should be presented on a bar or line graph. Line graphs show patterns or trends over time; pie charts display components of the whole. Comparisons of two or more variables may be displayed on bar graphs, stacked bar graphs, and line graphs. A Pareto chart is a special type of bar graph or histogram that plots the most frequently occurring category on the left to the least frequently occurring category. This type of chart facilitates a clear identification of the most significant factors to be addressed in solving the problem. The type of data that are available and the purposes of the statistical analysis will help the HIM professional determine the type of graph to use. Many computer software programs can facilitate data display.

Interpretation is the process of reviewing collected and displayed data and drawing valid conclusions that can lead to a decision. Toward that end, the HIM practitioner should ask questions such as these:

- Do the data fairly represent the group being evaluated or monitored?
- Is the sample size appropriate?
- Are the data valid?

Developing conclusions regarding the data and reporting the findings are also the responsibility of the HIM professional. Follow-up studies may be undertaken if previous outcomes indicate the need.

Health Care Facility Statistical Terminology

There is increasing emphasis on the standardization of health statistics for the purpose of generating valid intrafacility and interfacility comparisons and analyses. Health care facilities typically define a service area as a "care unit," each with its own assigned beds. Comparisons can then be made among units in various locations in the facility. The HIM professional's consistent use of standard terminology and reporting methods will lead to more valid and reliable statistical results. Most health care facilities that provide inpatient services have their census reports computerized, but the reports must still be manually verified. The census reports are maintained by the admission, discharge, and transfer (ADT) system.

The following terminology is consistent with the *Glossary of Health-care Services and Statistical Terms,* published by the American Health Information Management Association.[4]

Census: The number of inpatients-residents present in the health care facility at any given time. (For example, 434 patients were in the facility at midnight.)

Daily census: The number of inpatients-residents present at the census-taking time each day, plus any inpatients-residents who were both admitted after the previous census-taking time and discharged before the next census-taking time. (For example, on April 18, the health care facility rendered care to 225 inpatients and 5 additional patients who were both admitted and discharged during the 24-hour period since the previous day's tally was taken; therefore, the daily inpatient census was 230.)

Inpatient-resident service day: A unit of measure denoting the services received by one inpatient-resident in one 24-hour period. (For example, on November 3, the health care facility rendered 326 inpatient service days of care.)

Total inpatient service days: The sum of all inpatient service days for each of the days in a specified period of time. (For example, the total number of inpatient service days for the month of November was 9,820.)

Length of stay (LOS): The number of days an inpatient-resident stayed in the facility, counted from admission to discharge. (Facilities typically count the day of admission and not the day of discharge so that a patient admitted on Monday and discharged on Thursday would have stayed three days.)

Total length of stay: The sum of the days' stay of any group of inpatients-residents who are discharged during a specified period of time—also referred to as discharge days. (For example, the total length of stay for 150 patients discharged in May was 540 days.)

Health Information Management

Other terms that have accepted definitions for statistical purposes include *hospital patient, hospital inpatient, hospital newborn inpatient, medical staff unit, medical care unit, special care unit, adjunct diagnostic or therapeutic unit, occasion of service, hospital outpatient, emergency outpatient unit,* and *encounter.* These and other terms related to health care facility statistics are defined in the *Glossary of Healthcare Services and Statistical Terms,* which is contained in the *Basic Healthcare Statistics for Health Information Management Professionals* by Karen Youmans.[5] Another useful source is the American Hospital Association's *Hospital Statistics,* the result of its annual survey of more than 6,200 hospitals.[6]

In some facilities, daily census reports are maintained according to organized clinical service as well as nursing unit or bed location. Thus for each service the computerized daily statistical report shows the number of patients who were admitted directly or by transfer and the number of inpatient service days.

All statistical data should be reviewed periodically so that obsolete or unused data are no longer collected. Because health care facility administration sets the pattern for data collection, the HIM professional should be aware of a need for new data that are related to newly developed activities in the facility. In addition, because needs for statistics can change, health information systems should be organized for flexibility.

Facilities may gather statistics for which there is no mutually agreeable definition among various institutions. Such data are useful only to those particular institutions and to persons who are aware of the limitations of the definitions. Such data may be useful for internal operational purposes.

Health Care Facility Rates

This section presents some sample statistical computations of selected health care facility rates and ratios. A basic principle underlying all of the rate formulas is the concept of *actual versus possible.* The number of times that an event actually occurs is the numerator of the fraction, and the number of times that an event could possibly occur is the denominator. A ratio is a comparison of one thing with another, such as the number of patients per registered nurse on duty, or 1:10.

In addition to the rates shown in this section, health care facilities collect more detailed information to complete various reports for organizations such as the Joint Commission, the AHA, and many state hospital associations. The AHA requests that member and nonmember institutions participate in its annual survey of hospitals. This survey compiles information on facilities and services, beds and utilization by inpatient service, total health care facility beds and utilization, financial data, and information on personnel. The nonconfidential data items are then used to generate national statistical data on health care facilities.

Average daily inpatient census

$$= \frac{\text{total inpatient service days for a period (excluding newborns)}}{\text{total number of days in the period}}$$

Example:

$$\frac{2{,}100 \text{ inpatient days}}{30 \text{ days}} = \text{average of 70 inpatients}$$

Bed occupancy ratio

$$= \frac{\text{total inpatient service days for a period} \times 100}{(\text{number of available beds}) \times (\text{number of days in the period})}$$

Example:

$$\frac{6{,}975 \text{ patient days} \times 100}{(250 \text{ beds}) \times (31 \text{ days})} = 90.0\%$$

Average length of stay (LOS)

$$\frac{\text{total LOS of patients discharged, including deaths, excluding newborns} \times 100}{\text{total discharges, including deaths, excluding newborns}}$$

Health Information Management

Example:

$$\frac{2{,}068 \text{ patient days}}{550 \text{ discharges, including deaths,}} = 3.7 \text{ days}$$

550 discharges, including deaths, excluding newborns

Cesarean section rate

$$= \frac{\text{number of cesarean sections performed} \times 100}{\text{number of deliveries, including cesarean sections}}$$

Example:

$$\frac{28 \text{ cesarean sections} \times 100}{200 \text{ deliveries, including cesarean sections}} = 14.0\%$$

Mortality Rates

Mortality, or death rates, are calculated as they are an outcome that indicates the quality of care provided by the health care facility.

Health care facility mortality rate (may or may not include newborns)

$$= \frac{\text{number of deaths of inpatients} \times 100}{\text{number of discharges, including deaths}}$$

Example:

$$\frac{6 \text{ inpatient autopsies} \times 100}{320 \text{ discharges}} = 1.88\%$$

Maternal mortality rate

$$= \frac{\text{total number of direct maternal deaths} \times 100}{\text{total number of obstetrical discharges, including deaths}}$$

Example:

$$= \frac{2 \text{ maternal deaths} \times 100}{1{,}500 \text{ obstetrical discharges}} = 0.13\%$$

Neonatal mortality rate

$$= \frac{\text{number of newborn deaths} \times 100}{\text{number of newborn discharges, including deaths}}$$

Example:

$$\frac{4 \text{ newborn deaths}}{431 \text{ newborn discharges}} \times 100 = 0.93\%$$

Fetal death rate

$$= \frac{\text{number of intermediate and/or late fetal deaths}}{\text{number of live births, and intermediate and late fetal deaths}} \times 100$$

Example:

$$\frac{3 \text{ intermediate and/or late fetal deaths}}{300 \text{ births (total of live births, and intermediate and late fetal deaths)}} \times 100 = 1.0\%$$

Autopsy Rates

Fetal death autopsies are generally excluded in calculating autopsy rates, but newborn deaths and autopsies are generally included.

Gross autopsy rate

$$= \frac{\text{total number of inpatient autopsies}}{\text{total inpatient deaths}} \times 100$$

Example:

$$\frac{9 \text{ inpatient autopsies}}{25 \text{ inpatient deaths}} \times 100 = 36.0\%$$

Net autopsy rate

$$= \frac{\text{total number of inpatient autopsies}}{(\text{total number of inpatient deaths}) - (\text{unautopsied coroners' or medical examiners' cases})} \times 100$$

Example:

$$\frac{9 \text{ inpatient autopsies}}{(25 \text{ inpatient deaths}) - (7 \text{ unautopsied coroners' cases})} \times 100 = 50.0\%$$

Health care facility autopsy rate, adjusted

$$= \frac{\text{total number of health care facility autopsies} \times 100}{\text{number of deaths of health care facility patients whose bodies are available for autopsy}}$$

Example:

$$\frac{(9 \text{ inpatient autopsies}) +}{(2 \text{ emergency room death autopsies})} \times 100 = 55.0\%$$
$$(25 \text{ inpatient deaths}) - (7 \text{ unautopsied coroner's cases}) +$$
$$(2 \text{ emergency room death autopsies})$$

Vital Statistics and Records

Health records are the source documents for much of the information that is needed for birth, death, and fetal death certificates, which in turn are used for each state's vital record system. The HIM department may be responsible for preparing birth and fetal death certificates, as well as for transmitting the information to the registrar of vital records.

The National Center for Health Statistics of the U.S. Public Health Service prepares standard birth, fetal death, and death certificates that serve as models for use by individual states. The states use these model certificates to develop their own certificates and regulations regarding vital records. A state's health data center or division of vital statistics maintains the necessary information on preparing and registering vital records. The handbooks pertaining to a state's certificates can be obtained from the registrar of vital records in the state department of health, or the handbooks for the model certificates can be obtained from the U.S. Government Printing Office. The handbook from the federal government contains model certificates only because each state certificate is different. HIM professionals must be completely familiar with the regulations in their states so that correct procedures are followed. Every HIM department should have copies of the procedural handbooks that detail the registration of births, deaths, and fetal deaths.

HIM professionals must be aware of the importance attached to the prompt and accurate completion of these legal forms. Patient identification data and medical certification information on death certificates and fetal death certificates are completed by the health care facility and the attending physician, and the rest of the information is completed by the funeral director. Copies or worksheets of these forms are typically kept in the record for future reference. Some states require the health care facility to maintain a register of births and deaths. The register provides readily accessible information that can be obtained without referring to the patient health record.

Quality Control

The HIM department is responsible for the accuracy and reliability of collected data, whether in the preparation of vital statistical documents or in the computation of health care facility rates (discussed earlier in the chapter). Computerization of various statistical operations does not eliminate errors, because errors can occur in the inputting process or in the use of the statistical data that are generated from the computer. Clerical errors can always occur, as well as errors in abstracting. Edit checks should therefore be performed on a regular basis for all statistical applications. Because the data have many uses, it is vital that they be reliable and accurately reflect the care that is rendered by the facility for a given period. In addition, data format and data display techniques should be reviewed to determine whether the most effective methodology is being used. Routine quality control studies in both manual and computerized statistical systems ensure that the necessary collection of information is accomplished as efficiently and effectively as possible.

Duplication of effort in the statistical collection of data can be avoided when the HIM professional communicates with other departments and shares information on the data items of interest and their related purpose. In addition, criteria can be developed to determine the need for collecting various data items. Modifications often are needed, depending on the requirements of agencies such as the Joint Commission or the state department of health.

CONCLUSION

The expertise of the HIM professional is crucial to the success of the facility's health information system. Because of his or her knowledge and skills related to health care databases and database management systems, medical classification systems, clinical information flow, and medicolegal issues and security, it is essential that the practitioner be involved in the implementation and management of the health information system. The HIM professional directs or participates actively in all phases of operations related to collecting, storing, retrieving, analyzing, evaluating, and disseminating health data.[7]

REFERENCES

1. *Joint Commission on Accreditation of Healthcare Organizations, 2002 Comprehensive Accreditation Manual for Hospitals* (Oakbrook Terrace, Ill.: Joint Commission, 2002).
2. Ibid.
3. AHIMA, Practice Brief, "Designing a Data Collection Process," *Journal of AHIMA* (May 1998).
4. Karen Youmans, *Basic Healthcare Statistics for Health Information Management Professionals* (Chicago: AHIMA, 2000).
5. Ibid.
6. American Hospital Association, *Hospital Statistics* (Chicago: AHA).
7. Mervat Abdelhak, ed. *Health Information: Management of a Strategic Resource*, 2nd ed. (Philadelphia: W.B. Saunders, 2001).

BIBLIOGRAPHY

Duffy, P. "Data Dictionaries: An Overview." *Journal of AHIMA* 68, no. 2 (February 1997): 30.
Martin, T., and Fuller, S. "Components of the CPR: An Overview." *Journal of AHIMA* 69, no. 9 (October 1998): 58.
Shakir, A. "Tools for Defining Data." *Journal of AHIMA* 70, no. 8 (September 1999): 48.

CHAPTER 10

Quality Management and Performance Improvement

Linda S. Kiger

Health care facilities have long been involved in evaluating their quality of care through activities such as morbidity and mortality reviews and retrospective audits. Yesterday's quality improvement initiatives—known as quality assurance (QA) programs—have evolved into today's continuous quality improvement (CQI) and total quality management (TQM) programs. (The outdated term *quality assurance* is now considered a misnomer because it erroneously implies that quality can be guaranteed.)

Briefly, CQI consists of ongoing efforts to improve processes and performance in order to achieve consistently better results. CQI thus involves monitoring, evaluating, and adjusting processes. In contrast, TQM is a broader-based, more inclusive program in which the entire organization—beginning with top-level management—is committed to, and responsible for, quality improvement. TQM requires that every employee believe that there is always room for improvement and that every individual is responsible for contributing to improvements. TQM includes CQI and the management systems that are involved in such activities—for example, communication, education, and commitment of resources. Unlike quality assurance, which tends to be externally driven, focused on individuals and projects, and concerned with assigning blame and meting out punishment, TQM is internally driven; it focuses on processes and on the needs of the customer, and it rewards innovation.

Quality management (QM, also known as *quality assessment*) typically refers to activities such as utilization management (an evaluation of the health care facility's appropriate use of resources), risk management (the effort to control safety and financial threats to health care facilities), infection control, operative and other procedure review, clinical pertinence review, blood usage review, and medication use review. QM activities include work performed by various health care committees and the medical staff, as well as that of other professional staff from various facility departments. Some facilities have a separate QM or performance improvement department; others assign the responsibility to a section or unit of the HIM department.

Underlying the continuous assessment and improvement of quality care and the shift from QA to CQI are the standards of the Joint Commission on Healthcare Organizations. This chapter examines major requirements of the Joint Commission and those of the National Committee for Quality Assurance (NCQA), provides a brief survey of various approaches to quality assessment, and looks at the role of the HIM professional in quality assessment and improvement.

OVERVIEW OF JOINT COMMISSION STANDARDS ON PERFORMANCE IMPROVEMENT

The Joint Commission has been involved in formal quality assessment and improvement for many years—from the days of the first medical audits through its establishment of current standards for improving organization performance. Joint Commission standards require that health care facilities maintain an ongoing performance improvement program that monitors, evaluates, and improves the quality of care at the facility. The standards state that there must be a "planned, systematic, organization-wide approach to process design and performance measurement, assessment, and improvement."[1] Thus the Joint Commission requires an organization to improve continuously through the commitment and active involvement of its leaders. The facility must set priorities for assessment and improvement activities, select relevant indicators for monitoring purposes, and attend to customer orientation and feedback. The overriding purpose of all Joint Commission requirements is to ensure that the health care facility systematically works to improve its performance and takes appropriate action with regard to the assessment findings.

The Joint Commission's current standards for improving an organization's performance emphasize the following points:

- Activities are collaborative and interdisciplinary.
- New or modified processes are well designed.
- Data are collected to monitor the stability of existing processes, identify opportunities for improvement, and identify changes that lead to improvement and sustain improvement.
- Data are aggregated and analyzed on an ongoing basis.
- Improved performance is achieved and sustained.[2]

Monitoring performance through data collection is at the heart of performance improvement. Data collection focuses on

- Process, particularly those processes that are high-risk, high-volume, or problem prone
- Outcomes
- Targeted areas of study
- Indicators
- Other gauges of performance, including

  Clients' and others' needs, expectations, and feedback

  Results of ongoing infection control activities

Safety of the environment

Quality control and risk management findings

- Dimensions of performance (that is, efficiency and timeliness) that are important to a process or outcome[3]

Aggregating and analyzing data transforms data into information. Data analysis should answer certain questions, including these:

- What is our current level of performance?
- How stable are our current processes?
- Are there areas for improvement?
- Was the strategy to stabilize or improve performance effective?

According to the Joint Commission, "the goal is to develop an analysis process that incorporates four basic comparisons: with self, with other comparable organizations, with standards, and with best practices."[4] Statistical techniques (run charts, control charts, and so on) are used to analyze data. Intensive assessment must be implemented when undesirable variations are detected in the analysis process. Specifically, intensive assessment must occur when a sentinel event occurs, as well as for all confirmed transfusion reactions, all significant adverse drug reactions and medication errors, all major discrepancies between pre- and postoperative diagnoses, and adverse events during anesthesia use.[5]

CONTINUOUS QUALITY IMPROVEMENT

The performance of CQI activities requires either a model or systematic method, as well as personnel who are trained to gather, analyze, and report on data. The sections that follow provide a brief overview of some currently used major models and the roles played by the QM department in the performance of CQI.

CQI Models

Joint Commission standards do not require the health care facility to adopt any particular management style or to subscribe to any particular school or theory of CQI. Nor do the standards mandate any specific tools or methodologies for improving quality. Many models and methods for performing the CQI process are described in the literature and are currently in use. Among them are the Plan-Do-Check-Act (PDCA) cycle, the Joint Commission Ten-Step Method, and benchmarking.

The PDCA Cycle. W. Edwards Deming developed one of the earliest CQI models. The Deming cycle, more commonly known as the PDCA cycle, involves the following four major steps:

1. Planning change by studying a process, deciding what could improve it, and identifying data to help

2. Testing the proposed change by data stimulation or small-scale trial

3. Checking the effects by studying the results and modifying the planned changes if necessary

4. Acting to improve the process by implementing change[6]

This process has the advantage of being simple and easy to learn. In addition, an ongoing procedure resolves one problem as it begins to investigate another.

The Joint Commission Ten-Step Method. The Joint Commission's ten-step process, created to help organizations make the transition from quality assurance to CQI, is another valid approach to monitoring quality improvement activities. Many facilities still find that the ten-step process adequately serves their needs. The steps require the facility to do the following:

1. Assign responsibility for the department or service's monitoring and evaluation activities.

2. Delineate the scope of care or service that the department provides.

3. Identify the most important aspects of that care or service.

4. Identify indicators of quality and appropriate nature for the recognized important aspects of care.

5. Establish thresholds for evaluation (maximum allowable error rates).

6. Collect and organize relevant data, compare the data with the pre-established criteria, and analyze the findings.

7. Evaluate care. (Compare actual rate to thresholds.)

8. Take action to improve care and services.

9. Assess the effectiveness of actions and maintain the gain.

10. Communicate results to affected individuals and groups.

Process Improvement Model. This model comes from the former Quality Management Section of AHIMA:

1. List and prioritize improvement opportunities.

2. Define improvement project and QI team.

3. Analyze process problems.

4. Speculate as to causes of problems.

5. Test assumptions.

6. Identify root causes.

7. Consider alternative solutions.

8. Design solutions and controls.

9. Address resistance to change.

10. Implement solutions and controls.

11. Check performance.[7]

Benchmarking. Benchmarking is the comparison of the performance of one organization with another that is known to be excellent in that area. Comparisons can also be against regional and national standards.[8]

The Quality Management Department and CQI

Data collection for any of the previously described CQI models is performed by QM department personnel or by individuals in other areas who have been trained to retrieve data, such as HIM professionals. Regardless of the model used to perform CQI, pertinent data must not only be collected but also analyzed and displayed so that those involved can assess their significance. The HIM professional is responsible for providing excellent data, recognizing that accessible and accurate health information is essential to the organization's success. Reliable data enable the facility staff to answer questions, better understand processes, and ultimately make better decisions for improved patient care. Health care purchasers are also demanding data that illustrate a facility's ability to deliver high-quality health care.

Each department or service is responsible for documenting the effectiveness of its QM activities and for reporting such endeavors to the facilitywide program. QM department staff members, who may be titled QM systems analysts, quality support coordinators, or clinical data specialists who perform the QM coordinating functions, should, in turn, be responsible for demonstrating that the overall facility process is functional and effective. The data must be consolidated and reported to the medical staff, to administration, and to the health care facility's board of directors. Such reports include the following elements:

- A description of the study
- The method used to identify significant processes
- The department or service involved
- The person assigned to perform the study

- The data sources used

- The cause of the variations, if any

- Any corrective action undertaken

- The person who implemented the action

- The timetable for implementation

- Whether the issue was improved

- Plans for a monitoring procedure

- Plans for restudy

The persons involved must remember that QM activities are confidential matters. Special procedures must be followed to avoid any violation of health care facility policies on the handling of confidential information.

Computerized health information systems have affected and enhanced quality assessment and improvement reporting. The statistical results of quality indicator data are documented in spreadsheet software programs; the preparation of graphs and other statistical presentations is facilitated with the use of computer programs. Software programs are also used to conduct tracking and monitoring and to prepare comparative databases and outcome profiles. On-line data entry enables reports to be run at any time to demonstrate the facility's compliance with various standards. The HIM professional may be instrumental in selecting appropriate systems and software to collate and display data.

The quality review process has consistently moved away from retrospective examinations toward a concurrent review of clinical indicators to improve patient care. To that end, reviews now focus on clinical outcomes and clinical indicators relative to the effective quality management of patients and resources.

CLINICAL OUTCOME REVIEW, CLINICAL INDICATORS, AND QUALITY MANAGEMENT REAPPRAISAL

Outcome measures review the result or product of the patient's encounter with the system. A quality indicator is an objective, quantifiable measurement that targets events or patterns of events that may be suggestive of a problematic process or behavior. There are two basic types of indicators: (1) a sentinel event and (2) patterns of events that are revealed in aggregate data. A sentinel event is an infrequent, undesirable occurrence of such significance that it warrants comprehensive investigation—for example, loss of limb or function. The other type of indicator—patterns of events—consists of typical problems that, when they occur frequently, require a focused review. Such problems include, for example, surgeries that often run longer than planned. The problem could be caused by faulty scheduling, the actions of a particular operating room team, a piece of equipment, or a variety of other occurrences.

The QM outcome focus is global. Based on the philosophy that all processes can be improved, QM review information is used to study and improve the quality of care at a facility. The objectives, scope, organization, and effectiveness of the activities used to assess and improve quality should be evaluated at least annually and revised as necessary. In doing so, the facility can evaluate changes that have occurred as a result of QM efforts, examine quality indicators, assess the impact of the process on patient care and clinical performance, and make adjustments in the QM system.

As health care facilities complete the transition from QA to CQI, TQM, and performance improvement, HIM professionals face interesting challenges. A significant amount of material has been published regarding CQI and TQM, and the resources available in this area are many. Quality improvement thinking will be a major part of health care facility operation for the near future.

THE NEXT EVOLUTION IN ACCREDITATION AND THE HEALTH PLAN EMPLOYER DATA AND INFORMATION SET

In 1997, the Joint Commission approved new requirements for participation in the accreditation process for hospitals and long-term care facilities. The requirements apply to performance measurement and support the integration of performance data into the accreditation process. Hospitals and long-term care facilities select and enroll in one or more performance measurement systems (the providers must hold a Joint Commission contract) that meet the commission's initial requirements for inclusion in the accreditation process. The Joint Commission named this accreditation process ORYX: The Next Evolution in Accreditation.[9]

The goal of ORYX is to ensure a more thorough, continuous, and comprehensive accreditation process. The system moves beyond standards evaluation to the assessment of outcomes. Organizations select and report on clinical measures. Failure to do this can lead to a loss of accreditation. A health care organization's performance data are compared only to its own data and to the data from other health care organizations that have selected the same measures in the same system. During the initial phase, the number of measures increased to six over a period of four years. The second phase includes the identification and use of core measures, that is, standardized performance measures that can be applied across accredited health care organizations in a particular accreditation program. In May 2001, the Joint Commission announced the four initial core measurement areas for hospitals: (1) acute myocardial infarction, (2) heart failure, (3) community-acquired pneumonia, and (4) pregnancy and related conditions. Hospitals began collecting core measure data for patient discharges on July 1, 2002.[10]

The HIM professional should be very involved in selecting a performance measurement system that meets this Joint Commission initiative. The system should measure data that are relevant to the organization's population, have the ability to adapt to future expectations, and be sufficiently stable over time.

Health Plan Employer Data and Information Set (HEDIS) is a set of standard performance measures designed to provide purchasers and consumers with information necessary to compare the performance of managed health care plans. The National Committee for Quality Assurance sponsors, supports, and maintains HEDIS. The current version of HEDIS (HEDIS 2001) is outcomes- and results-oriented. It looks at how well patients function in their daily lives and measures health plans' successes at improving functional status.[11] Data are collected using claims information, health record review, and a combination of the two.

Performance measures include the following elements:

- Effectiveness of care
- Access and availability of care
- Satisfaction with care
- Health plan stability
- Use of services such as well-child visits and inpatient utilization
- Cost of care
- Informed health care choices
- Health plan descriptive information

HEDIS is an internal measurement tool that is useful for benchmarking, identifying areas for quality improvement, and enhancing physician profiling. As the health data content expert, the HIM professional can work to improve data collection practices in an effort to facilitate all the performance measurement elements. The HIM professional adheres to national coding guidelines and uniform data collection practices that, in turn, provide solid data for HEDIS reporting.

PROFESSIONAL PRACTICE STANDARDS FOR HIM

The American Health Information Management Association (AHIMA) has published *Professional Practice Standards for Health Information Management Services* since 1984; the standards were revised most recently in 1998. Standards also exist for the fields of ambulatory care, long-term care, and behavioral health. In the area of QM systems, the standards suggest that HIM professionals "develop and coordinate systems to promote continuous improvement of the quality of services rendered, the appropriate utilization of organizational resources, and the management of risks to consumers and health care providers."[12] The rationale is that the health record provides the basis for assessing patient care services. The HIM professional has managerial and technical skills to support the QM and CQI programs, as well as skills in utilization management (UM) and risk management (RM). The HIM professional can demonstrate this professional standard by participating in the development of QM policies and procedures, as well as by organizing, aggregating, and displaying QM data for the medical staff, administration, and other health care facility departments.

Another function of the HIM professional, as supported by the professional practice standards, is to coordinate data collection systems that are related to the utilization and quality assessment of the health care services provided by the facility. The manager might develop systems to promote the continuous improvement of services throughout the organization or conduct cost benefit analyses for QM, UM, or CQI activities. The HIM professional may function as a clinical data analyst, a clinical data systems manager, or a data quality manager. In these roles, the individual is responsible for outcomes management and data integrity, as well as for providing information for decision making and strategy development, participating in high-level analysis projects such as outcomes research, or establishing procedures for newly integrated services and entities. To accomplish all these tasks, the individual must be skilled in data management. The HIM professional must provide strategic leadership in this area of expertise.

CQI AND QA IN HIM

In the same way that a health care facility attempts to improve the quality of its services through a facilitywide continuous quality assessment program, the HIM department can establish a quality assessment program to improve the quality of services that it performs and provides. A CQI program for the department should follow the same basic steps as the program for the entire health care facility.

The HIM professional first assesses current department activities and determines how they relate to a CQI program. The focus of CQI, as well as

TQM, is to ensure that the entire organization, beginning with top-level management, becomes committed to, and responsible for, quality improvement. Quality is most appropriately expressed in terms of customer needs. When the need is stated to be "accuracy in the codes that are submitted for payment of claims" or "accuracy in the transcription of dictation," systems can be developed for quality checks of the work performed.

A department CQI program includes selecting the policy, topic, or procedure that is to be evaluated, developing evaluation criteria or standards, monitoring data, evaluating results, determining the causes of the variations or problems identified, developing and implementing corrective action, conducting follow-up on the corrective action undertaken, and reporting to the administration and the staff of the HIM department. The department director and staff develop the objectives for the QM activities and set standards so that an objective review of the activity can take place. Standards are either qualitative or quantitative, and they can be determined through work sampling, direct time studies, or published staffing methodologies.

After the standards for an activity are established, procedures are developed to measure the actual practice in the department against the standards. This measurement discloses any variations in specific areas. When variations exist, the cause as well as corrective steps or recommended solutions must be determined. In addition, the individuals who are responsible for corrective action or implementation of a solution must be clearly identified. Follow-up monitoring will provide information on the effectiveness of the corrective action that is undertaken.

In the implementation of a CQI program, employee orientation to the philosophy of CQI and TQM is important, as is inclusion of employees in the development of standards for their own activities. Because TQM is not a program but a set of philosophies and a different way of approaching issues, it is crucial that TQM have the support of department and facility staff. Setting objectives and standards and conducting ongoing evaluations require a time commitment from the department staff and its director, who must plan for the cost of implementing a department CQI program. Clearly, the cost savings that result from improving processes outweigh the costs of establishing a program. Verification checks for accuracy, consistency, and uniformity of data that are recorded and coded for databases, statistical record systems, and for use in QM and performance improvement activities are a regular part of the health record abstracting process.

Other benefits of a CQI program include its usefulness in studies of internal department operations such as accuracy in filing a paper record in the permanent file, accuracy of the chart tracking system, accuracy in the filing of loose material in a paper record, and accuracy in coding and abstracting procedures. By establishing standards for activities and measuring current employee activity against the standards, a CQI program becomes an excellent cost-containment tool for improving department operation and the quality of services rendered. As the concepts of TQM and CQI are an integral part of the operation of hospitals and other health care facilities, the data collection, analysis, and display skills of the HIM professional are crucial.

RISK MANAGEMENT

Risk management (RM) is the process of identifying, evaluating, and eliminating or controlling risks that pose safety threats to patients or financial threats to health care facilities. A facility's RM program should be closely related to its QM program. Some facilities create separate RM departments; others incorporate RM efforts in the duties of other groups, such as the HIM department. In risk management, a financial and statistical approach is used to focus on patients, nurses, physicians, other health care professionals, and ancillary employees. A health care facility often employs a risk manager who evaluates the interaction of all risk components and assesses the risks for the facility.

The successful operation of an RM program depends on commitment by the facility's administration. Only with the support of high-level administrators can the risk manager become involved in all areas of the facility that may contain or generate risks. The risk manager should also have access to incident reports, employee accident data, and so forth.

The HIM professional assists the risk manager in identifying, evaluating, and eliminating or controlling risks. The health record is an important screening tool for identifying information related to facility risks. The facility may choose to perform generic screening or occurrence screening to identify risks. Occurrence screening involves the concurrent or retrospective identification of physician and facility-related adverse patient occurrences. The term *generic screening* is sometimes used for this process because the criteria used may be applied to all patients and are not tied to a diagnosis or procedure. For example, adverse reactions to medications, transfusions, and anesthetics could be reviewed.

UTILIZATION MANAGEMENT, CASE MANAGEMENT, AND DISCHARGE PLANNING

Utilization management is a broad term that encompasses the review of appropriate medical intervention and analysis of a facility's efficiency in providing necessary services in the most cost-effective way. UM focuses not only on assessing a patient's need for continued stay in the health care facility but on evaluating the appropriate level of care as well. A UM program includes documentation of the utilization review plan, as well as the actual utilization review process. The HIM professional must play an instrumental role in coordinating the health care facilities' UM, QA, and performance improvement programs. The HIM professionals' expertise in statistics and data analysis makes this a strong area of practice.

The Joint Commission defines *utilization management* as "the examination and evaluation of the appropriateness of the utilization of a [health care facility's] resources."[13] Utilization reviews may be prospective—that is, before any services are rendered—or concurrent with the rendering of patient care. Criteria measuring the intensity of service and severity of illness are used. The patient's medical condition is compared with standard criteria to reflect his or her need for hospitalization or need for continued hospital-level care. Health care facilities are also required to review support services with regard to appropriateness, clinical necessity, and timeliness. Examples would be radiology, medical laboratory, or pharmacy.

The utilization review plan should identify instances in which non-physician health care professionals could participate in the utilization review process. The plan should be reviewed annually and revised when appropriate.

The HIM department is often involved in concurrent reviews and in reviews and initial screenings of patient records at admission and at designated continued-stay review dates. Using written, measurable criteria and length-of-stay norms approved by the medical staff, HIM professionals perform the initial and follow-up screening of inpatient records for the health care facility.

A case management approach and performance of early discharge planning are also components of the effective utilization management of health care facility resources. In case management, all aspects of a patient's care, including his or her rehabilitation potential, the medical services being rendered, and the patient's potential ability to return to an appropriate productive employment situation, are reviewed. Coordination among various disciplines and the clinical management of patients in specific case groups for episodes of care, is vital to a successful case management approach. Case managers must determine the necessary and appropriate resources for the provision of desired patient outcomes through such activities as monitoring patient variances from clinical pathways, identifying quality and utilization issues, preparing trend reports on variances, and beginning early discharge planning.

The HIM professional who functions as a case manager may help educate all members of the health care team regarding accreditation standards or reimbursement changes. HIM professionals may be involved in team conferences with an employer-sponsored private review program. He or she can also communicate with third-party payers or peer review entities regarding clinical and fiscal information for financial optimization, and evaluate and analyze patient outcomes to identify opportunities for improvement.

Discharge planning should begin early in the patient's hospitalization. To facilitate discharge as soon as an acute level of care is no longer required, the Joint Commission's patient assessment standards require that discharge planning be initiated as early as the physician makes a determination of the need for such activity.

CONCLUSION

Effective functioning by the HIM professional in the area of utilization management or performance improvement is integral to the facility's success in these areas. The health record data used in case management, risk management, discharge planning, and other aspects of QM and performance improvement must be accessible and accurate. Whatever approach or system is used by the health care facility, health record data lie at its core. The HIM professional must manage and coordinate a health information system to provide data that enable a health care facility to continually improve its quality of patient care. Embracing CQI and performance improvement thinking will promote excellence in HIM.

REFERENCES

1. Joint Commission on Accreditation of Healthcare Organizations, *2002 Comprehensive Accreditation Manual for Hospitals* (Oakbrook Terrace, Ill.: Joint Commission, 2001).
2. Ibid.
3. Ibid.
4. Ibid.
5. Ibid.
6. Abdelhak, Mervat, ed. *Health Information: Management of a Strategic Resource,* 2nd ed. (Philadelphia: W.B. Saunders, 2001).
7. Brown J. *The Healthcare Quality Handbook* (Pasadena, Calif.: JB Quality Solutions, 2001).

8. Elliott, C., et al. *Performance Improvement in Healthcare* (Chicago: AHIMA, 2000).
9. Zeglen, M. "Accreditation Requirements for ORYX: The Next Evolution in Accreditation," *Journal of AHIMA* 68, no. 6 (1997): 20–25.
10. Joint Commission on Accreditation of Healthcare Organizations, *2002 Comprehensive Accreditation Manual for Hospitals* (Oakbrook Terrace, Ill.: Joint Commission, 2001).
11. National Committee for Quality Assurance, *HEDIS 2001* (Washington, D.C.: NCQA, 2000).
12. AHIMA, *Health Information Management Practice Standards: Tools For Assessing Your Organization* (Chicago: AHIMA, 1998).
13. Joint Commission on Accreditation of Healthcare Organizations, *2002 Comprehensive Accreditation Manual for Hospitals* (Oakbrook Terrace, Ill.: Joint Commission, 2001).

WEB SITES

www.hcqa.org

www.ahima.org

www.jcaho.org

CHAPTER 11

Preservation
of Health Records

Linda S. Kiger

T his chapter examines the preservation of health records. The length of time that health records should be archived and the format in which they should be retained (original, microfilm, optical CD-ROM, or other) are complex issues. In selecting the retention program most consistent with the health care facility's operation, the facility is guided by its needs for patient care and by existing state laws, as well as research and legal requirements. Guidelines should be developed that specify the information to be archived, the storage medium in which it is maintained, and the length of time the information is to be retained.

RETENTION OF HEALTH INFORMATION

The Institutional Practices Committee revised the American Hospital Association's statement on record retention titled "Preservation of Medical Records in Health Care Institutions" in 1990. It states, in part:

> The primary purpose of the medical record is to document the course of the patient's illness and the treatment received. Although the medical record is kept for the benefit of the patient,

physician, and the health care institution, it is the property and responsibility of the health care institution to safeguard and preserve its content.[1]

The length of time that health records are retained depends on the purposes for which the records are being maintained. These purposes include patient care needs, clinical or scientific research needs, and assessment activities pertaining to the quality of patient care. An additional consideration is the possibility of future patient litigation. The Conditions of Participation for health care facilities involved in federal programs require that medical records and radiology service films, scans, and images are to be retained for a period of at least five years.[2]

Although most states legislate retention requirements that health care facilities must follow, in some jurisdictions the facilities are not required by law to preserve their records for any given length of time. In these states, the appropriate period of retention is affected by the statute of limitations for bringing a legal action for an injury or breach of contract. In most states, the period of the applicable statute of limitations is less than ten years. However, in many states the statute of limitations requires that an action for personal injuries sustained by a minor be exercised within a few years after he or she attains majority status (that is, reaches the age of eighteen).

Health care facilities should not preserve health records that duplicate other permanent official records. Keeping records solely for proving birth or age, residence, citizenship, or family relationships serves no useful purpose. Because health care facilities are seldom asked to produce health records that are more than ten years old, the AHA recommends that complete patient medical (or health) records be retained, either in the original or reproduced form, for ten years after the most recent date of patient care. This holds true in the absence of legal considerations and unless destruction of the records is specifically prohibited by statute, ordinance, regulation, or law.

After ten years, the following information, at a minimum, should be retained:

- Dates of all visits
- Admission and discharge dates
- Names of responsible physicians
- Records of diagnoses and procedures, including any applicable physician attestations
- History and physicals (H&P forms)
- Operative and pathology reports
- Discharge summaries (clinical résumés)

The complete health records of minors should be retained for the period of minority status, plus any applicable period that is specified in state statutes relating to the retention of records of minors or the statute of limitations. Complete health records may be retained longer when requested in writing by any of the following individuals:

- An attending or consulting physician of the patient
- The patient or someone acting legally on the patient's behalf
- Legal counsel for an individual having an interest affected by the health records

The adoption of a record retention policy, as suggested by the AHA statement on preservation, could reduce the previous period of retention by the health care facility. Therefore, the AHA recommends that any new policy be developed with the full knowledge and participation of the medical staff, legal counsel for the facility, and any past or present liability insurance carrier affording coverage during any time that the affected records were created.

The AHA statement also recommends that any new policy on record retention be communicated to all appropriate individuals and organizations, as suggested by the facility's legal counsel. Either the lesser period of retention should be restricted to subsequently completed health records or the general application of the lesser period of retention should be delayed for a reasonable length of time to allow requests for deferred destruction to be received.

AHIMA issued a revised practice brief in January 1999 regarding the issue of retention of health information. The actual brief lists all component state associations with laws or regulations pertaining to retention, and it should be referenced for a particular state guideline. Any one of the following means may determine the length of time that health records should be preserved: health care facility policy, the statute of limitations or other legal requirements, the policy statement of the AHA, the needs of the medical staff, and other factors specific to the individual health care facility. HIM professionals should work with appropriate facility personnel in developing, implementing, and controlling a retention system that safeguards the physical records, including their medical and health data, for future retrieval.

DESTRUCTION OF PATIENT HEALTH INFORMATION

Although the HIM professional must carefully consider the type of information to maintain, its duration, and the means by which to preserve it, another issue to consider is the development and implementation of a record destruction policy. A carefully planned record retention policy includes destruction dates that relate to the various state record retention guidelines. Documents that are retained beyond the destruction date occupy valuable storage space and cause needless expense. (However, records that relate to litigation or any open investigation or audit should not be destroyed.) AHIMA's practice brief on the destruction of patient health information includes the following recommendations:

- Records should be destroyed so that there is no possibility of reconstructing any information.

- If a facility makes a decision to destroy computerized data, it should develop methods of destruction that obliterate the data permanently and irreversibly.

- Pulverization should be employed as an appropriate means of destruction for laser disks that are used in write-once-read-many (WORM) document imaging applications.

220   Health Information Management

- The method of destruction should be reassessed annually.

- The destruction should be documented, including the date, method, description of the disposed record series, inclusive dates covered, a normal course of business statement, and signatures of all persons involved.

- Destruction documents or certificates should be maintained permanently.

- If destruction services are contracted, the contract should include such things as method, confidentiality requirements, and indemnification from unauthorized disclosure.[3]

The procedure for handling and storing confidential information before it goes out for storage or destruction must be communicated to all departments. Final destruction can be accomplished with one of many methods, from shredding or recycling to incineration. If an outside company is used, the storage firm or service bureau should ensure that the transportation, storage, and destruction of the records is handled not only according to the retention guidelines but with strict attention to the control of costs and confidentiality as high priorities.

MICROGRAPHICS OR MICROFILMING

When a health care facility intends to preserve its health records and does not have the space available to keep all records in the paper format, micrographics, also called microfilming, is one appropriate method of preservation. The terms *microfilm, microform,* and *microimage* can be applied to any information, communication, or storage medium that contains images too small to read without magnification. Before records are microfilmed, the HIM department may need to contact the state health department, the state hospital licensing agency, or other appropriate state regulatory agencies concerning microfilming requirements, regulations affecting the retention of health records, and provisions regarding the use of microfilm as evidence in court actions. The facility's legal counsel should also be consulted in decisions that involve microfilming health records. Counsel will be aware of specific microfilming regulations that affect operations in the state. Some states require authorization or approval from the regulatory agency before the original records may be destroyed. The HIM department should be familiar with any legal ramifications that arise from microfilming and future use of the film. When space is at a premium, the facility may be able to obtain permission to microfilm records earlier than state regulations would otherwise permit.

The health care facility may elect to carry out the microfilming process entirely with its own personnel, contract for microfilming services with an outside company, or use a combination of in-house and commercial processing. For example, the facility's in-house personnel might prepare records for a service company to microfilm. Choosing to perform the microfilming process at the facility requires a large investment in equipment and maintenance, as well as the personnel costs of operating the equipment. Regardless of the system that is selected, the original health records must not be destroyed until HIM personnel have reviewed the microfilm for quality and accuracy.

When the facility's officials decide to enter an agreement with a microfilm service bureau (usually a private business that provides micrographic and record management services), they should consider the following characteristics of the vendor before awarding a contract:

- Range of services offered
- Type or condition of the equipment to be used
- Expertise of the service's staff
- Past performance of the service in similar applications
- Level of understanding regarding application requirements
- Ability to provide high-quality services within the time allotted
- Cost of services
- Quality and speed of service requests
- Likelihood of adherence to industry standards

- Records management service options
- Disaster contingency program, if any

Microfilming can be performed annually, semiannually, or quarterly. When space needs are acute and records are microfilmed within two to five years after patient dismissal, a quarterly schedule is often desirable. The activity of the records is the key factor in determining the retention and microfilming schedule. The facility may choose to microfilm old records at the same rate that new records enter the system.

Microfilm storage and retrieval systems are designed to enable users to locate a desired image from among thousands of others. The health care facility can select from various methods and media to house the microfilm, including those in the following list:

- *Roll film:* Roll film, which may contain several hundred records on each roll, is suitable for serially numbered records if requests for the records are few. Roll film is the most economical medium; it works well with extremely old records or records of deceased patients. Its major disadvantage is that the confidentiality of other patient records may be jeopardized when a particular record is requested in court and the entire roll is submitted. Retrieval is also time consuming unless a computer-assisted retrieval system is also used.

- *Cartridges and cassettes:* Cartridges and cassettes are designed for users who want the advantages of roll film without the inconvenience of manual film handling. Cartridges and cassettes offer more flexibility; however, they are more expensive than roll film. They may be used in file systems where files are frequently referenced.

- *Microfiche:* Microfiche (a sheet of film that contains multiple microimages) has the advantage of easy and direct access to information because all of the information on a patient appears on an individual sheet rather than on a long roll. Some microfiche can be updated—a feature that allows patient information that is microfilmed later to be housed with the original record. Microfilm jackets of transparent acetate can be used to hold microfilm in flat strips. New images can be added to the jacket or old images deleted. Each jacket can hold about seventy document pages, depending on the reduction ratio that is used.

• *Computer output microfiche:* COM is a process by which computerized digital data are converted to readable text or graphic information on microfilm without first creating paper documents. The computer holds magnetic tapes that contain data for generating reports. COM has several applications, including computerization of a master patient index (MPI). COM takes information that is stored in a computer or on magnetic tape, translates it into readable form, and displays it on a computer display screen. As this process eliminates the steps of filming, developing, and loading the microfilm jacket, it offers significant savings over other methods.

• *Computer-assisted retrieval:* CAR is a method of locating and retrieving documents using computer indexes. It is used with roll or jacket microfilm to create an automated document storage and retrieval system. CAR combines the qualities of high storage capacity, permanence, security, legal acceptability, and other benefits of microforms with the technology of computers for rapid index retrieval. CAR systems provide rapid reference to randomly filmed records using computerized indexing and cross-referencing.

Microfilming is still a viable option for the preservation of health records. The nature of the application, the level of complexity involved in finding a desired record in the present system, and the number of people who need access to the information are some of the considerations related to the choice of a micrographics system.

From a practical point of view, microfilm is a stable storage medium in humanly readable form. The HIM professional may select microfiche, roll film, or COM and may use a CAR system. Each has advantages, but careful advance planning and research are required in choosing the correct medium.

OPTICAL DISK OR CD-ROM STORAGE

HIM departments also use optical disk or CD-ROM storage as a method of health record retention. Optical disk storage uses a laser to etch data onto a prepared surface of permanent material, also called a laser disk. Optical disks can store vast amounts of paper information on a single disk. A single CD-ROM can store thousands of documents, and retrieval of any one of those documents can be accomplished in seconds. The system is used with a stand-alone personal computer, a local area network (LAN), or a large central system or network. Data are entered into the system either concurrent with the patient hospitalization or at discharge.

System components include a scanner to digitize the documents; a workstation that includes a central processing unit, monitor, and keyboard; a "jukebox" that holds and retrieves optical disks as they are requested; a file server to retrieve images for users on the system; and optical character scanning devices to index data automatically. A printer is needed for output, or information can be faxed to a remote location when required.

An optical disk system includes the following benefits:

- Easy and quick access to the stored health record
- Round-the-clock availability of the health information to authorized users without support staff assistance
- Simultaneous access by multiple users to the health information
- Security that can control unauthorized access
- Improved quality of patient care due to ease of access to previous health information
- Space savings over paper-based records
- Productivity gains due to a decrease in the amount of time spent moving records from one location to another
- Increased use of computer technology

- On-line availability of information (the system can incorporate data from different sources as it is electronically created at many sites within the facility)
- Ease of performing database searches for specific information that has been indexed

The primary disadvantage of an optical disk system is the cost of implementation. Also to be addressed are costs for training, education, and standardization, as well as legislative issues. Although the system is compatible with a computerized record system, security and confidentiality are major issues of concern. HIM professionals should provide the balance that is necessary between ease of access to the health information and the privacy of that information.

Off-site storage of records—a choice currently being used by some facilities—is not necessary with an optical disk storage system. Monetary savings in this area, as well as in copying records requested after discharge, are possible with an optical disk system. The computer system prints copies of records as requested, and employee time that is currently spent photocopying records is saved. The timely capture, storage, distribution, and processing of information are achieved with electronic imaging.

CONCLUSION

Overall, the health care facility needs an effective record retention and retrieval program in order to access information for patient care and financial, research, statistical, and educational purposes. The HIM department must be able to provide accurate, complete, and useful health care data from active and inactive patient records. The department is responsible for providing this information in the most efficient and effective manner possible. The computer-based patient record will change the storage media so that electronic storage and image-based records will be the most prevalent methodology. One role of the HIM professional in the future will be that of document and repository manager. He or she must possess current knowledge in this area and should be a leader in identifying the systems that are most appropriate for the particular facility.

REFERENCES

1. American Hospital Association, *Preservation of Medical Record in Health Care Institutions* (Chicago: AHA Institutional Practices Committee, 1990).
2. *Medicare Conditions of Participation for Hospitals,* 42 Code of Federal Regulations, 482.24(b)(1) and 482.26(d)(2) (Washington, D.C.: Government Printing Office, 2001). On-line, available at www.access.gpo.gov
3. AHIMA, Practice Brief, "Practice Guidelines for Managing Health Information," *Journal of AHIMA* 67, no. 1 (January 1996). On-line; available at www.ahima.org

CHAPTER 12

Location, Space, and Equipment Requirements

Linda S. Kiger

The HIM department is a vital component of the health care facility. Personnel in that department remain in constant communication with the admissions or registration departments of the regular inpatient units, ambulatory care units or satellites, and emergency care units. In addition, personnel in the HIM department communicate clinical information to the business office for claims processing and receive notices of discharges and reports of diagnostic and therapeutic procedures from ancillary departments.

This chapter examines the logistical, service, and equipment requirements of the HIM department. Major factors such as health record filing and processing needs are reviewed, along with the requirements for maintaining databases such as the MPI and space requirements for HIM personnel. The chapter closes with an overview of factors to consider when planning a new HIM department. Although the scope of this coverage does not permit a detailed analysis of all factors to consider, a checklist of major considerations is provided in Figure 12.1.

Figure 12.1. Checklist of Logistics, Services, and Equipment Requirements

- What services are the responsibility of the HIM department?

- What is the extent of computerization in the department?

- How do the records and data flow to and from admitting, the nursing units, the emergency department, the business office, ambulatory clinics, the financial department, and other areas?

- What is the best means of efficiently capturing health information, whether the record is paper or electronic?

- Is telemedicine technology used to transmit information from one site to another?

- How will reports of diagnostic or therapeutic tests and treatments be integrated into the health record—in a paper record or computer-based record?

- Will records of readmitted patients be automatically sent to the nursing unit on patient admission, or will they be furnished only on request?

- What type of area will be maintained for record completion by responsible parties?

- Who will be authorized to have access to the HIM department for record retrieval if the department is not continuously staffed around the clock?

- Are ambulatory care patient records and emergency records maintained in a unit record and therefore filed in the same chart folder with the inpatient record?

- What is the relationship between record and information systems management with the health care institution's satellite facilities?

- Do the filing and storage systems that are used provide for easy retrievability of records?

- How many internal requests for information are received for patient care studies?

- What is the health care facility's plan for implementation of the computer-based patient record?

Figure 12.1. Continued

- Will optical disk technology be used for record storage?

- What is the preservation period for the health record? How long is the record retained in active files within the department? Will inactive records be retained in hard copy, and, if so, where will they be filed? Are inactive records currently stored on microfilm, paper, optical disk, magnetic tape, or other media?

- What is the facility plan for record destruction?

- Which department services are outsourced?

- What is the long-term systems plan for the electronic medical record? Will new optical hardware be attached to the department's microcomputers (or personal computers)? What is the network system?

- What application software is currently used for coding, DRG assignment, statistical data collection, tumor registry, quality assessment, utilization management, chart tracking, and so on?

- How many requests are received for release of health record information to sources outside the health care facility in the form of correspondence, telephone calls, subpoenas, or court orders?

- What information security systems are in place to protect the confidentiality of both paper-based and computer-based health information with regard to HIPAA privacy and security requirements?

- Which clinical and financial database is necessary for integration with the health care facility's information system?

- Is the department director responsible for any other departments, such as admissions or registration or the business office?

- Is there decentralization of any record functions, such as having record analysis and completion done at the nursing unit?

- Has a universal chart order been established?

- To what extent do outside parties such as quality improvement organizations and surveyors utilize the department?

LOGISTICAL, SPACE, AND EQUIPMENT CONSIDERATIONS

Every day, medical staff members complete or reference health records in the HIM department. Ensuring the prompt completion of, and ready access to, health records requires that the HIM department be located in an area that is accessible to the medical staff and in close proximity to the admissions or registration, emergency, and business departments. In addition, admitting or nursing personnel need access to the department if it is not open around the clock. Security surveillance to safeguard health record information and information systems when the department is closed is also a consideration when reviewing locations for the HIM department.

Space allocation is determined by the departmental services provided, the equipment and systems used, and the daily workload handled. Although services vary among health care facilities, services and tasks considered in allocating space include those in the following list:

- Maintenance of the file area

- Master patient indexing

- Record assembly and analysis

- Coding and abstracting

- Release of information

- Medical transcription

- Department management

- Record completion

- Departmental functions regarding the following elements:

  Quality assessment

  Clinical pertinence review

  Cancer registry

  Outside record review by representatives of various organizations (for example, a state quality improvement organization) or outside contracted services

The Permanent File

Record file management includes the receipt, filing, retrieval, and dissemination of records from both active and inactive file areas. Open-shelf file units are the most commonly used storage method for health records. High-density, movable, open-shelf filing equipment can be electrically operated for access and require less space than other open-shelf filing units. File manufacturers and suppliers offer shelving with various widths and options to maximize storage and filing space. Although traditional filing cabinets may have some usefulness, the need for this type of equipment has declined with the increase in information maintained within the facility's computer system.

Movable file units that rest on tracks are one potential space-saving option. However, a disadvantage of this system is the limited access to files, which may be an issue in a busy department. Automated filing systems are available for easy record retrieval. Such a system may bring requested records to the appropriate person by entering some basic data. Although automated filing systems can save time, increase efficiency, and be used with all types of media, they have the disadvantage of being costly to implement.

Space allocations usually allow 36 inches for aisles between filing units, although 30 inches can be used when there is a crucial shortage of floor space. Main aisles must be at least 5 feet wide. Standards set by the Occupational Safety and Health Administration (OSHA) determine some space allocations.

The Unit-Numbering System. The unit-numbering system implies that the patient receives the same number for each admission or visit to the health care facility. Therefore, if a unit-numbering system is used, the department director must ensure that adequate space is provided on the shelf for the growth of records due to readmissions and repeat clinic visits. Reviewing data from previous years is the best predictor for future space requirements. The director should determine the average size of his or her facility's health record in order to project the linear filing inches that will be required for the next five to ten years.

Active and Inactive Record and File Locations. The terms *active* and *inactive* are used in referring to both the health record and file locations. A health record is typically classified as active when the last discharge or visit date is within three to five years of the current date. Active records are maintained in readily accessible files that are referred to as *active files*. If there were a sharp decline in readmissions between three and five years, the decision might be made to maintain records for only the past three years in the active file area.

Statistical data on the rate of readmissions should be maintained and used in planning for current and future space needs. These data provide needed information for department management and for facility administration. Maintaining data on readmissions that occur within designated time periods, such as one month, six months, one year, and five or ten years from the date of last discharge provides valuable data for the health care facility's information management system. Data accessed by utilization management, for example, are useful in reviewing readmissions that occur at specific intervals. A facilitywide CQI team may identify and explore any problems that are identified in the data.

Inactive records are less often retrieved and refiled. Therefore, these files may be located in an area that is less accessible than that for active files. Inactive files may be microfilmed or put on optical or magnetic disks to save space. Microfilming and computer storage also provide easy accessibility. Space requirements depend on whether the microfilming is performed in-house or by an outside company. In addition, space consideration should address the type of equipment that is necessary to store and read the storage media and to convert this medium into paper copy.

The length of time that a record must be retained in original or miniaturized form varies from state to state. Each state hospital association can provide information on the state's legal requirements for record retention. Two useful references are the American Hospital Association's statement on record retention, *Preservation of Medical Records in Health Care Institutions,*[1] and the AHIMA practice brief "Practice Guidelines for Managing Health Information."[2]

The MPI

The MPI—the permanent database file that identifies all patients who have been admitted or treated by the health care facility—is the key to locating patient records and is a crucial data storage source for the facility. (Recall that data in this database are maintained after record destruction.)

The amount of space to be allocated for the MPI depends on the type of equipment or system to be used for immediate identification of current and past patients by name, address, birth date, health record number, and possibly by other identifying data. Traditionally, manual index cards or electrical rotary files were used in health care facilities. Now the computerized MPI is becoming more common, saving space and, more important, facilitating the retrieval of information. With terminals located throughout the health care facility, a computerized index makes identification information available to all departments.

Record Assembly and Analysis

Workspace is needed in the HIM department when records are assembled there and subsequently analyzed for completeness. During this process, staff members generate various forms and documents that are used in incomplete record control and chart tracking. When a HIM professional performs record assembly and analysis at the nursing unit, less space is needed, of course, in the department. However, a designated work area must exist at the nursing unit for the HIM professional.

Coding and Abstracting

Systems for coding and abstracting can be manual, computerized, or a combination of the two. When coding (or encoding) is computerized, space needs include an area for the computer and its component parts. A manual system requires space for the health records, coding books, reference materials, and abstracting supplies. Whether a computerized or manual system is used, space should be allocated to store the indexes that are generated from the data.

Release of Information

The health care facility's release-of-information function may be handled with internal or outsourced staff or both. The workstation should include space for the computers, printers, duplicating equipment, telephones, fax machine, and any other equipment that is necessary to carry out this function satisfactorily. The workstation may be located near the entrance to the department or near a service window that is convenient for public access. Requests for information may be made in person by the patient or by another person with authorized access to the record. The request may also be made by phone from another health care facility or from a physician's office for continued patient care.

Medical Transcription

Transcription department systems have gone from electronic typewriters and loose cassette tapes to fully integrated word-processing databases and digital dictation systems. As such, the transcription service is able to access the dictation system, the patient demographic system, and other systems in transcribing medical dictation.

The HIM professional should become thoroughly knowledgeable about the myriad computerized solutions to the process of producing voluminous, timely patient care reports. Selection of an integrated suite of medical document management options requires knowledge of dictation, transcription, document replication, and distribution. One solution is for a health care facility to maintain its own hardware and a network-based environment so that data can be shared among all users. Another is to employ voice-recognition technology that transmits the spoken word to a database for immediate review or printout, thus eliminating the need to transcribe dictation. In such a digital dictation system, the caregiver verbally records patient information, and it is then electronically documented using medical transcription technology. The department director should weigh the advantages and disadvantages of such a system from a variety of vendors.

In processing medical dictation, a department can use a medical transcription service rather than fulfill this function in-house. When an outside service is used, the department director should work with the service to establish and maintain standards for quality and confidentiality.

Department Management

The HIM professional who manages the department should have an office with sufficient space for conducting supervisory conferences and management-level meetings. Meetings conducted with physicians, administrators, department employees, or others require privacy. Other management personnel within the department may also require individual offices, or the floor layout can provide for shared offices among the supervisory staff.

Physician Record Completion

A work area for physicians to use in completing health record documentation is typically located adjacent to the HIM department. It should be accessible and quiet and provide tools for complete access to the health care facility's clinical information system. A shelving area may be necessary to house the incomplete records. Space must also be available for medical staff members and others to conduct any reviews of health records for research and other data-gathering and analysis activities.

Quality Assessment, Utilization Management, and Other Functions

Although quality assessment, utilization management, and cancer registry are sometimes separate departments, they are often components of the health care facility's HIM department. The inclusion of these functions in the HIM department directly affects its space and equipment considerations. Space requirements vary with the size and responsibilities of the staff, as well as with the degree of computerization of the various functions assigned to the department.

The HIM department also needs a designated work area for use by various outside parties who have a legitimate need to review or utilize patient records. Such individuals include representatives from quality improvement organizations, third-party payers conducting reviews and audits, and contractors performing coding services or other outsourced activities. Attorneys also request access to original health records and may perform their review in the department. Physicians may perform record reviews within the department.

The HIM professional should develop, maintain, and control an information management system that is accessible to all who are authorized to use it. Adequate space and equipment to support this access must be provided for optimum performance of the facility's health information system.

Additional Space and Equipment Considerations

In addition to the space requirements previously described, other functions of the department warrant comment and consideration. For example, space may be needed for equipment that transports volumes of records to decentralized units around the health care facility. In addition, an area may be needed within the department for sorting records and storing reference materials and supplies.

Space for Employee Desk Arrangements. To provide adequate workspace, 60 square feet per employee is suggested for desk arrangements. When optimum configurations and space allocations are not possible, the department director must solve space problems through innovative designs that use workstations and equipment. The HIM professional should be familiar with the principles of layout and functional planning to design the workspace for maximum operational efficiency.

Computerization and Space Requirements. The extent of computerization within an HIM department directly affects its space requirements. The department may be linked to the health care facility's mainframe computer, or a local area network may be in place. The LAN links personal computers within a limited area, such as a floor or a building. Computerization extends from the MPI through all units within the department. Optical disk or magnetic disk (or tape) storage can be used for storing health records. Savings in space, microfilming costs, personnel time, and copying are made possible by using such computerized methodologies (see Chapter Eleven). However, cost may prohibit the adoption of the very latest technologies.

Workload and Space Requirements. The workload of the department is an important determinant of its space and equipment requirements. Workload is based on the volume of information that is processed on a daily, weekly, monthly, and yearly basis. The extent of information that is processed per day, week, or month in each service area of the department should be determined, including the elements that follow:

- Number of new admissions added to the MPI and the extent of its utilization
- Number of discharges processed
- Volume produced by the word processing or transcription section
- Number of requests for release of health record information
- Number of records being abstracted and coded and the corresponding number of data items
- Number of records being retrieved, disseminated, and refiled
- Any expected changes in workloads

The workload that is determined for one year may change during the next year when the facility's corporate plan includes expansion or downsizing of the patient care facilities. Hence, in the strategic planning process the department director projects future needs of the health care facility's information system.

Space limitations caused by an increase in workload can require operating one or more service areas for sixteen to twenty-four hours per day. In larger health care facilities, three or more department service areas are typically in continuous, round-the-clock operation.

Support Areas

The services of the health care facility's education and training department should be available to the HIM department. The HIM department, like others in the facility, should have access to classrooms or meeting rooms for in-service training programs, video conferencing, teleconferencing, and staff meetings. Provisions should be made to allow the HIM department to schedule the use of this space.

SYSTEM AND EQUIPMENT SELECTION

The director of the HIM department should always use the best methods and the latest technology to generate the flow of health information. He or she should also select products that meet the health care facility's need for efficient production and high quality at reasonable cost. Before equipment and systems are selected, however, the features to be assessed should be itemized. The questions listed in Figure 12.2 should be addressed.

Technological changes continue to occur at a rapid rate, and equipment and systems offer new and improved features every year. For example, more sophisticated optical imaging, bar coding, and voice recognition systems continue to be developed. The patient record of the future will be computer-based. However, in today's health care facilities, it is unlikely that most HIM departments will receive the funding that is necessary to computerize all HIM functions at once. Decisions for equipment and systems therefore need to be made consistent with which functions are automated and when.

Understanding the direction of technological development in hardware and application software is crucial to the systems and equipment decision making of HIM professionals. As a case in point, department directors must recognize that, with the total integration of clinical information systems, data may conceivably be shared throughout the facility's system using a mainframe and individual PC workstations that are networked. LANs will be established in increasing numbers in the health care environment. Choosing a software package that operates on hardware that is becoming obsolete could become be a costly mistake.

In general, the equipment and systems needs of the facility's HIM department are affected by the following factors:

- The department's functions and staffing levels, which may allow certain types of equipment to be used over long periods and may require a good communication and dispatch system for reduced staffing on evenings and weekends
- The department's choice of a centralized or decentralized system for inpatient and outpatient records or a separate location for transcription, which may require transportation and communication systems and equipment
- The number of emergency visits to the health care facility and clinics, which require health records to be retrieved and dispatched immediately, and the number of scheduled visits to the clinics, which require the record to be retrieved and dispatched before clinic hours
- The integration of the health care facility's clinical and financial management systems, including databases that are maintained

An integrated information system can focus on quality-of-care and patient care data and can provide information on the medical staff, payers, payment trends, and other financial details. The purpose of such linkage of clinical and financial information is to provide data immediately to those who need it. The data may be needed for patient care or for some other aspect of effective health care facility operation.

Figure 12.2. Equipment and Systems Features Checklist

- Will this system or equipment meet the needs associated with current and projected workloads?

- What are the system's space requirements?

- Will additional space be needed if the workload increases?

- Will the amount of paperwork be reduced? If so, by what percentage?

- Can information or data be changed or updated easily and quickly, as appropriate?

- Will data be secure from unauthorized access?

- Does the system or equipment have the necessary flexibility for integration with other systems or equipment in the department and health care facility?

- Can this system or equipment perform a variety of tasks or applications?

- Is this system or equipment cost-effective from the standpoint of reduced personnel time or increased productivity?

- What are the warranty period and provisions, the costs for various types of maintenance, and the response time for service calls?

- Is a back-up system needed for downtime?

- How much training time is needed for employees? Will the vendor provide the training? Are training materials available?

- Will the vendor provide support services in the development of applications? If so, what is the associated cost?

- What is the reputation of the vendor or manufacturer? Will the company provide references from other users for an overall evaluation of system, equipment, or services? Are other facilities that use the equipment satisfied with its performance? Is the vendor's base of customers large enough to provide reliable data? Can you see in operation what the vendor has promised?

- What is the purchase price? Is leasing an option?

Health Information Management

Figure 12.2. Continued

- Does the vendor's system operate on a hardware platform that is consistent with the criteria of the health care facility? Is it a nonproprietary hardware platform? This becomes important in integration of different vendors' systems.

- Does the vendor offer a pathway of automation? Is there an option to add, at a reasonable cost, modules that will share the same hardware and the same mainframe interface?

- Is the vendor showing financial stability by successfully selling the product and reinvesting generated profits into research and development for that product?

- Does the vendor offer user-group meetings to accept enhancement suggestions?

PLANNING FOR A NEW DEPARTMENT

The HIM professional who is involved in planning a new department has the monumental task of developing an integrated clinical data management system that meets the needs of the health care facility. This integrated system involves the collection of data from the following systems within the health care facility or department:

- The admitting, discharge, and transfer system
- The MPI
- The incomplete records management or record tracking system
- The record reservation or request system for records pulled for various purposes (such as clinic appointments or special studies)
- The appointment scheduling system
- The dictation system
- The abstracting-grouping-encoding system

- The release-of-information system
- The medical transcription or word processing system

Integrated clinical data management has many benefits. For example, it provides quality assessment personnel with data for individual and aggregate review and monitoring and the evaluation of facilitywide activities. It also provides data for such functional areas as infection control and utilization review. Such integration enables the health care facility to develop and implement strategies that affect the quality of care, the cost of high-quality care, and the efficiency with which the care is provided.

The HIM professional is the most logical individual to develop the clinical data management system because of his or her expertise and knowledge of documentation requirements, retrieval systems, data analysis, and clinical data interpretation. This knowledge should encompass the computer applications of health information. Up-to-date technological equipment must be purchased to continually improve and broaden the services provided by the HIM department.

The progressive HIM professional should build a computer-based patient record system and department and do so with a concern for patient confidentiality and an insistence on principles of standardization of the health information that is collected and maintained throughout the facility. The HIM professional will eventually become the manager of health information in a paperless environment.

CONCLUSION

At a time of significant change in the profession, the HIM professional should be involved in all aspects of planning relative to department logistics, including location, space allocation, and equipment selection. The HIM department and the information it contains should be accessible to many but restricted from others. Space considerations should reflect not only health care facility growth but the possibility of downsizing. Equipment decisions are significantly affected by the computerization of the department and the short- or long-range plan for the computer-based patient record.

REFERENCES

1. American Hospital Association, *Preservation of Medical Records in Health Care Institutions* (Chicago: AHA Institutional Practices Committee, 1990).
2. AHIMA, Practice Brief, "Practice Guidelines for Managing Health Information," *Journal of AHIMA 70*, no. 6 (June 1999).

WEB SITES

www.aha.org

www.ahima.org

www.osha.org

AHIMA POSITION STATEMENT

Privacy Officer

The American Health Information Management Association (AHIMA) recognizes the increased complexity of protecting patients' privacy while managing access to and release of information about patients and health care consumers. Credentialed health information managers are uniquely qualified to be the designated privacy official as required by the Health Insurance Portability and Accountability Act (HIPAA) through their academic preparation, work experience, commitment to patient advocacy, and professional code of ethics.

BACKGROUND

Health care is a service industry that relies on information for every facet of its delivery. Health information has value to the patient it describes, the provider it serves, the organization it supports, and to society, as it directs the health of the population. As a valuable asset it must be protected. In its primary form as the medical record of a unique individual, it must be safeguarded.

Privacy concerns grow as technology increases access to health information. Mental health, substance abuse, sexually transmitted disease, and now genetic information create a heightened awareness of the need for privacy. Documented cases of the use of health information to make decisions about hiring, firing, loan approval, and direct-to-consumer marketing have sensitized the public to the risks of sharing information with their health care provider. And ultimately, the erosion of trust between patient and provider may create the largest risk.

For years, states have written laws and regulations to protect their citizens' privacy by limiting release of information based on the requestor, the type of information, and the use of that information. Because of the complexity of the issue, the number of concerned parties, and the variety of health information, no two states have the same laws.

The federal government has tried over the last ten years to address the patchwork nature of state laws by developing comprehensive federal legislation but has failed to complete that task. In an effort to ensure that all citizens have a standard minimum protection, the Department of Health and Human Services has promulgated regulation under the authority of HIPAA to provide a universal floor of protection. However, the industry is already concerned with meeting this new minimal level.

To ensure the necessary leadership for compliance, the HIPAA-authorized regulation—The Standards for Privacy of Individually Identifiable Health Information, released in December 2000—requires that each health plan, health care clearinghouse, and certain health care providers must designate a privacy official who is responsible for the development and implementation of their policies and procedures relative to privacy.

Although the challenges are growing and new laws and regulations exist, health information management professionals have effectively managed the release of information in health care organizations for decades. Establishing policy, training staff, developing consents, releasing information, and documenting information use are key elements of the health information management role. Coursework that prepares health information managers to fulfill this role has long been included in the curriculum of all accredited health information management academic programs and is included in the certification examination for both registered health information administrators and technicians. Since its formation in 1928, AHIMA has supported its members in their efforts to protect patient privacy.

SUPPORT FOR THE POSITION

To maintain the privacy, confidentiality, and security of health information, AHIMA members assume a leadership role in compliance with state and federal laws, develop appropriate organizational initiatives, and exercise ethical decision making. Health information management professionals are uniquely qualified for this role because we

- Understand state and federal laws that apply to the use of health information
- Know the decision-making processes throughout health care that rely on information
- Understand the flow of information within health care organizations and throughout health care
- Apply health information management principles to information in all its forms
- Know the content of health information in its clinical, research, and business contexts
- Are aware of the technologies used to collect, access, store, and transmit information in all its forms
- Establish and recognize best practices in the management of privacy of health information
- Have managed the release of information function historically
- Have acted as the patient advocate relative to health information
- Live by a Professional Code of Ethics that is specific to maintenance of patient privacy

AHIMA SAMPLE

(Chief) Privacy Officer Job Description

Position Title: (Chief) Privacy Officer[1]

Immediate Supervisor: Chief Executive Officer, Senior Executive, or Health Information Management (HIM) Department Head[2]

General Purpose: The privacy officer oversees all ongoing activities related to the development, implementation, maintenance of, and adherence to the organization's policies and procedures covering the privacy of, and access to, patient health information in compliance with federal and state laws and the healthcare organization's information privacy practices.

Responsibilities:

- Provides development guidance and assists in the identification, implementation, and maintenance of organization information privacy policies and procedures in coordination with organization management and administration, the Privacy Oversight Committee,[3] and legal counsel.

- Works with organization senior management and corporate compliance officer to establish an organization-wide Privacy Oversight Committee.

- Serves in a leadership role for the Privacy Oversight Committee's activities.

- Performs initial and periodic information privacy risk assessments and conducts related ongoing compliance monitoring activities in coordination with the entity's other compliance and operational assessment functions.

- Works with legal counsel and management, key departments, and committees to ensure the organization has and maintains appropriate privacy and confidentiality consent, authorization forms, and information notices and materials reflecting current organization and legal practices and requirements.

- Oversees, directs, delivers, or ensures delivery of initial and privacy training and orientation to all employees, volunteers, medical and professional staff, contractors, alliances, business associates, and other appropriate third parties.

- Participates in the development, implementation, and ongoing compliance monitoring of all trading partner and business associate agreements, to ensure all privacy concerns, requirements, and responsibilities are addressed.

- Establishes with management and operations a mechanism to track access to protected health information, within the purview of the organization and as required by law and to allow qualified individuals to review or receive a report on such activity.

- Works cooperatively with the HIM Director and other applicable organization units in overseeing patient rights to inspect, amend, and restrict access to protected health information when appropriate.

- Establishes and administers a process for receiving, documenting, tracking, investigating, and taking action on all complaints concerning the organization's privacy policies and procedures in coordination and collaboration with other similar functions and, when necessary, legal counsel.

- Ensures compliance with privacy practices and consistent application of sanctions for failure to comply with privacy policies for all individuals in the organization's workforce, extended workforce, and for all business associates, in cooperation with Human Resources, the information security officer, administration, and legal counsel as applicable.

- Initiates, facilitates, and promotes activities to foster information privacy awareness within the organization and related entities.

- Serves as a member of, or liaison to, the organization's IRB or Privacy Committee,[4] should one exist. Also serves as the information privacy liaison for users of clinical and administrative systems.

- Reviews all system-related information security plans throughout the organization's network to ensure alignment between security and privacy practices, and acts as a liaison to the information systems department.

- Works with all organization personnel involved with any aspect of release of protected health information, to ensure full coordination and cooperation under the organization's policies and procedures and legal requirements.

- Maintains current knowledge of applicable federal and state privacy laws and accreditation standards, and monitors advancements in information privacy technologies to ensure organizational adaptation and compliance.

- Serves as information privacy consultant to the organization for all departments and appropriate entities.

- Cooperates with the Office of Civil Rights, other legal entities, and organization officers in any compliance reviews or investigations.

- Works with organization administration, legal counsel, and other related parties to represent the organization's information privacy interests with external parties (state or local government bodies) who undertake to adopt or amend privacy legislation, regulation, or standard.

Qualifications:

- Certification as an RHIA or RHIT with education and experience relative to the size and scope of the organization.

- Knowledge and experience in information privacy laws, access, release of information, and release control technologies.

- Knowledge in and the ability to apply the principles of HIM, project management, and change management.

- Demonstrated organization, facilitation, communication, and presentation skills.

This description is intended to serve as a scalable framework for organizations in development of a position description for the privacy officer.

NOTES

1. The title for this position will vary from organization to organization, and may not be the primary title of the individual serving in the position. "Chief" would most likely refer to very large integrated delivery systems. The term "privacy officer" is specifically mention in the HIPAA Privacy Regulation.
2. Again, the supervisor for this position will vary depending on the institution and its size. Since many of the functions are already inherent in the Health Information or Medical Records Department or function, many organizations may elect to keep this function in that department.
3. The "Privacy Oversight Committee" described here is a recommendation of AHIMA, and should not be considered the same as the "Privacy Committee" described in the HIPAA privacy regulation. A privacy oversight committee could include representation from the organization's senior administration, in addition to departments and individuals who can lend an organization-wide perspective to privacy implementation and compliance.
4. Not all organizations will have an Institutional Review Board (IRB) or Privacy Committee for oversight of research activities. However, should such bodies be present or require establishment under HIPAA or other federal or state requirements, the privacy officer will need to work with this group(s) to ensure authorizations and awareness are established where needed or required.

INDEX

by, 220–221; health information retention by, 217–220; health information storage options for, 221–226; risk management (RM) of, 212–213; statistical computations on rates of, 191–193; statistical terminology used by, 189–191; utilization management of, 213–214; vital statistics and records of, 47, 195–196

Health care facility registers: birth and death, 142; emergency department, 143; operating room, 143; patient, 141; special, 143–147

Health Information: Management of a Strategic Resource (Abdelhak), 37

Health record analysis: contemporary trends in, 97–102; issues in, 81; major steps in, 82–97; workspace set aside for, 235

Health record analysis steps: admission, discharge, transfer (ADT) reports, 82; assembling records, 82–84; documents/data reviewed, 88–97; qualitative analysis, 86–88; quantitative analysis, 84–86

Health record analysis trends: concurrent analysis, 99; electronic signature/other streamlining techniques, 99–100; focused review, 101–102; issues for record improvement, 97–99; simplified deficiency processing, 100–101

Health record forms (or chart order), 83

Health record structure: of discharged patients records, 37; integrated progress notes, 32–34; problem-oriented medical records, 34–37; source-oriented, 32; three options for, 31

Health records: abbreviations used in, 20; alternatives to unit record system, 41–42; ambulatory care, 24–26; assembling of, 82–84, 235; comparison of medical and, 1; content of, 19–20; emergency care included in, 26; federal/state requirements on content of,

97; functions of, 2, 45, 68; home care, 26–28; hospice, 29; Joint Commission/state content standards on, 20–21; kept by HMOs, PPOs, AHAs, 30–31; locations of active/inactive, 234–235; long-term care/rehabilitation, 28–29; maintenance/protection of, 5; mental health, 30; numbering/filing systems for, 105–126; professionals responsibilities for, 5*fig*–6, 68–69; release of information in, 236; rule compliance for reviewing/monitoring, 6; secondary data/disclosure of, 79, 129–147; structure of, 31–37; unit record system and, 38–41, 107–109, 233–234. *See also* EPR (Electronic patient record systems); MPI (master patient index); Patient health information; Patients

Health records preservation: destruction vs., 220–221; micrographics or microfilming for, 221–224; optical disk or CD-ROM storage of, 225–226; retention of health information and, 217–220

Health reports TAT (turnaround time), 87

HEDIS (Health Plan Employer Data and information Set), 208–209

HIM department: authority over unit record system by, 38; characteristics of effective numbering/filing systems used by, 105–106; director of, 14; functions of, 8; health record preservation options for, 221–226; health record responsibilities of, 5*fig*; health record used in, 1–2; integration of coded data produced by, 17; logistics, services, equipment requirements of, 230*fig*–232*fig*, 232–244; privacy officer of, 247–254; utilization management, case management, discharge planning role by, 213–215

HIM department logistics/space/equipment: checklist for, 230*fig*–232*fig*; computerization and space requirements,

238–239; employee desk arrangements, 238; management of, 237; medical transcription, 48, 236–237; for new department planning, 242–244; of permanent file, 233–236; physician record completion, 237; quality assessment and, 135–136, 179–212, 237–238; space and equipment considerations, 232; support areas, 240; system and equipment selection, 240–241, 242*fig*–243*fig*; utilization management, 213–214, 237–238; workload and space requirements, 239–240

HIM permanent file: assembly/analysis of records in, 81–102, 235; coding/abstracting of, 47–48, 122, 149–170, 235–236; locations of active/inactive records and, 234–235; release of information from, 236; space allocation/location of MPI (master patient index), 235; space allocations for, 233

HIM professional: AHIMA position on privacy officer, 247–249; career opportunities of, 10–11; department director position of, 14; educational requirements for, 11–13; job descriptions for, 13; knowledgeable about JCAHO standards, 10; mental health record documentation standards and, 30; practice standards for, 209–210; privacy officer, 247–254; relationships with other departments, 15–16; Vision 2006 on roles of, 14–15

HIM professional responsibilities: AHIMA on, 8–9; clinical database management as, 176, 177–178; for CQI and QA implementation, 210–212; database/statistical quality control as, 196–197; deficiency systems/follow-up activities, 85–86; EPR system data validation, 62–64; EPR system selection, 61–62; financial/information systems management, 16–17; health record responsibilities of, 5*fig*, 25–26, 68–69;

HEDIS implementation by, 209; to improve the documentation system, 101–102; ORYX: The Next Evolution in Accreditation and, 208–209; overview of, 8–10; qualitative analysis, 86–88; Vision 2006 (1996), 14–15

HIM Technology: An Applied Approach (Johns), 37

HIPAA Final Rule, 151

HIPAA (Health Insurance Portability and Accountability Act), 15, 59–61, 114, 182

HL7 (Health Level Seven), 75

HMOs (health maintenance organizations): health records kept by, 30–31; as managed care, 170

Home health care: records on, 26–28; standardized data set for, 184

Hospice records, 29

Hospital Statistics (AHA), 191

I

ICD-9-CM: coding research/cooperating parties and, 154–155; current application of, 152–154; described, 150, 151–152; DRG reimbursement and, 155–156; mental disorders and, 157–158; oncology and, 157; outpatient reimbursement and, 156–157; uniform hospital discharge data set in accordance with, 181

ICD-9-CM Coding Handbook (AHA), 154

ICD-9-CM Coordination and Maintenance Committee, 155

Image-based EPR systems, 51–54

Incidence, 188

Index for Radiologic Diagnoses, 158

Information-capture design: duplicating systems options and, 77–79; gathering facts to create tools for, 72*fig*; improving existing tools for, 73*fig*–74*t*; practice guidelines for, 67–69; principles of computer-view, 74–76; principles of, 76–77; principles of paper form design

Patients: analysis of history/physical examination of, 90–91; ICD-9-CM standards on reimbursement for outpatients, 156–157; informed consent of, 23; records of discharged, 37, 82, 89–90. *See also* Health records; Medical records

PCs (personal computer) networks, 125

PDAs (personal digital assistants), 64

PDCA (Plan-Do-Check-Act) cycle, 203

Performance improvement standards (JCAHO), 200–202

Phonetic filing system, 134*t*

Photocopying forms, 78–79

Physical examination record. *See* H&P (history and physical) examination

Physician index, 139

Physician orders analysis, 93–94

Physicians: medical record responsibilities by, 7; record completion by, 237. *See also* Medical staff

Physicians' Current Procedural Terminology (AMA), 159

"Pick list" program capability, 56

POMR (problem-oriented medical records): advantages and disadvantages of, 36–37; database component of, 35; described, 34; initial plan component of, 35; problem list component of, 35; progress notes component of, 35–36

Population, 185

PPOs (preferred provider organizations): health records kept by, 30; as managed care, 170

PPS (prospective payment system), 149, 151, 177

"Preservation of Medical Records in Health Care Institutions" (1990), 217–218

"Preservation of Medical Records in Health Care Institutions" revision (1999), 220

Prevalence, 188

Privacy issues: rule (HIPAA regulation) on, 59–60; Social Security numbering system and, 112–113. *See also* Confidentiality

Privacy officer: AHIMA job description of, 251–254; background information on, 247–248; support for, 249

Process improvement model (AHIMA), 204

Professional Practice Standards for Health Information Managements Services (AHIMA), 209

Progress notes analysis, 92–93

PROs (Peer Review Improvements), 179

Q

QA (quality assurance) programs, 199

QIOs (Quality Improvement Organizations), 179

Qualitative analysis: qualitative review checklist, 87–88; quality assessment study and, 86

"Quality Healthcare Data and Information" (1996 AHIMA), 163

Quality management department: clinical outcome review, clinical indicators and reappraisal by, 206–207, CQI and, 205–206

Quality management/assessment (QM): described, 200; HIM department logistics for, 237–238; HIM professional's role in, 210–212; MPI (master patient index), 135–136; new JCAHO accreditation requirements and, 207–209; performance improvement standards and, 200–202; QA, CQI, TQM programs for, 179, 199–200; statistical techniques, 196. *See also* CQI (continuous quality improvement)

Quality Services Demonstration Project, 164

Quantitative analysis of health records: deficiency follow-up activities and, 86; deficiency systems and, 85; overview of, 84–85

R

Radiological report analysis, 94–95

RBRVS (Resource-Based Relative Value Scale), 151, 162

Real-time transfer, 57

Total length of stay, 190
TQM (total quality management) program, 199–200, 211, 212
Tracking systems, 121–123
Transcription, 48, 236–237
Transfer records: analysis of ADT reports on, 82; analysis of summary in, 89–90; nursing documentation on, 95–96
Trauma registry, 145–146
2002 Comprehensive Accreditation Manual for Hospitals, 42

U

UACDS (Uniform Ambulatory Care Data Set), 179, 182
UHDDS (Uniform Hospital Discharge Data Set), 138, 179, 180–181
UHI (unique health identifiers), 113–114
UM (utilization management), 179
Uniform Ambulatory Care Data Set, 25
Uniform Data Set for Home Care and Hospice, 27–28
Unit numbering system: described, 107–108; HIM permanent file and, 233–234; manual/automated issuance of numbers, 108; procedures for error correction, 108–109; shelf requirements for records filing, 109
Unit record system: alternatives to, 41–42;

arrangement of information in, 39–40; benefits of, 40; content of, 38–39; described, 38; format of, 40–41
Universal chart order, 83–84
"Upcoding," 165
UPIN (unique personal identification number), 139, 180, 181, 183
U.S. Department of Health, Education, and Welfare, 180
U.S. Department of Health and Human Services (DHHS), 167
U.S. Public Health Service's National Center for Health Statistics, 154
Utilization management, 213–214, 237–238

V

Validity, 188
Variable, 185
Vision 2006 (1996), 14–15
Vital statistics records, 47, 195–196

W

WANs (wide area networks), 125
Weed, L., 34
WHO (World Health Organization), 151, 152

Y

Youmans, K., 191